MEDICAL CARE CAN BE DANGEROUS TO YOUR HEALTH

MEDICAL CARE CAN BE DANGEROUS TO YOUR HEALTH

A Guide to the Risks and Benefits

(Previously published as <u>Matters of Life and Death</u>)

Eugene D. Robin, M.D.

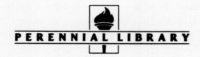

PERENNIAL LIBRARY

Harper & Row, Publishers
New York, Cambridge, Philadelphia, San Francisco
London, Mexico City, São Paulo, Singapore, Sydney

To my wife, Jane,
who provides poetry for this writer of prose

This book was published originally under the title *Matters of Life and Death* as a part of *The Portable Stanford,* a series of books published by the Stanford Alumni Association and later by W. H. Freeman and Company. It is here reprinted by arrangement with W. H. Freeman and Company.

First PERENNIAL LIBRARY edition published 1986.

Library of Congress Cataloging-in-Publication Data

Robin, Eugene Debs, 1919–
  Medical care can be dangerous to your health.

  Reprint. Originally published: Matters of life & death. New York : W.H. Freeman, c1984.
    1. Iatrogenic diseases—Popular works. 2. Health risk assessment. 3. Medical care. I. Title. [DNLM: 1. Iatrogenic Disease—popular works. 2. Medicine—popular works. QZ 42 R 655m]
RC90.R63   1986   362.1   85-45656
ISBN 0-06-097029-4 (pbk.)

86 87 88 89 90 MPC 10 9 8 7 6 5 4 3 2 1

Contents

Preface

The past 20 years have seen an unprecedented accumulation of medical knowledge. This has been accompanied by a growing and unprecedented disillusionment with the application of this knowledge to patient care. Dissatisfaction is expressed by increasing numbers of patients and is even shared by many doctors. In fact, when the doctor becomes a patient, his anxieties may be even more intense than those of a medically untrained person. At the very time that medicine has achieved a new pinnacle of formal progress, confidence in its relevance to patient welfare may be approaching a nadir.

This paradox has not gone unnoticed. Numerous publications deal with one or another of the perceived causes—economic, political, cultural, scientific, or societal. Most analyses have not directly challenged the system whereby medical knowledge is applied to patient care. This book, written primarily for the general public, makes such a challenge. It stems from my conviction that there are major but reversible flaws in the present system of medicine; that these flaws can be understood by most patients and potential patients; and that while waiting for medicine and society to correct these flaws, patients themselves can help minimize the risks of modern medicine.

I do not regard this book as heretical or myself as a heretic. I do believe in some things. I believe that the purpose of medicine is to help patients directly. I believe that we need more, not less, science in medicine, but it has to be better science and more closely linked to patient welfare than it is today. I believe that medicine can be markedly improved but that this improvement will not happen automatically. I do not regard myself as an iconoclast even if I succeed in smashing a few idols. Nor do I consider myself a medical nihilist. I have tried to provide constructive alternatives to those features of medical care I consider wrong or inadequate.

Nor am I a professional critic of medicine. Actually, I am a teacher and researcher. In my research, I am trying to unravel the mechanisms by which lack of oxygen affects genetic expression of cells—hardly a controversial area. I teach physiology and clinical management to undergraduate medical students, interns, residents, fellows, and physicians in practice. I tell them much of what I will tell you, with varying degrees of success. I am also a doctor, involved in the care of patients. I like to think that I do that better than I used to because I am more critical of myself and my colleagues than I used to be. I certainly feel more humble than I once did.

This book grew out of a series of teaching exercises for doctors that I have conducted during the past five years. Underlying those exercises and this book are certain assumptions:

· The goal of doctors should be to help patients as much as possible (hardly a revolutionary or world-shattering assumption).
· Much of what we doctors do is tangential to that purpose.
· Much of what we do is harmful.
· Many of the tangential and harmful aspects of medical care could be changed.
· We doctors should take the major responsibility for changing them.

Although there have been notable exceptions, on the whole the reception of these teaching exercises by other doctors has been surprisingly favorable. This encouraged me to believe that the material might be useful to nondoctors also. This book, then, is for everyone who is or might be a patient.

Many of the ideas I present in this book are not original with me, but I accept the responsibility and blame for whatever is wrong or harmful. Whatever else you may get from the book, I hope it will encourage you to evaluate more critically the opinions furnished by medical experts—my own included.

Many of the concepts developed in this book have not been subjected to experimental verification. For many of them it would not be possible to do so. You may consider this an important weakness in my argument. You will have to trust or reject my ideas on grounds of logic, intuition, or personal experience.

I have tried to be precise about facts, primarily because it is the right thing to do, but also because the book may be subjected to unusually close scrutiny. If any inaccuracies have escaped me, I apologize, but I hope that you will not be distracted by these from the main thrust of the book.

I have provided a glossary of terms, many of which you may already know. In my choice of what to include I have supposed that everyone knows a congenital disease is a disease one is born with. Not everyone may know, however, that congenital diseases are not always inherited (i.e., genetic in origin), but may be acquired in the womb; for example, as a result of a uterine infection or a drug given to the mother. Most everyone, I imagine, knows that a cardiologist is a heart specialist.

I have not provided a reading list because, in my opinion, the medical literature is imperfect and contradictory. Using it selectively to support my views would provide unjustified support and a sense of false erudition. This book deals with very fundamental attributes of medicine, and fundamentals are usually impossible to prove. In the last analysis, this book represents my own opinion, as it must.

I feel uncomfortable using "he" and "his" to include both women and men, but I could not find a solution that did not seem artificial and distracting. I hope that linguists will soon come up with a term that embraces both genders.

Though not specifically written as a textbook, this book can be used as a nontextbook textbook. You can even, if you choose, participate in a formal examination that will test what you may have learned while "studying" the text (see back of book for details). On the other hand, you may choose to read it casually in whole or in part. Whichever alternative you choose, I hope that you learn as much from the reading as I have learned from the writing.

Eugene D. Robin

Stanford University
September 1984

Acknowledgments

I am indebted to approximately fifty colleagues, patients, and friends, who read and commented on portions of the text in its various stages. I especially want to acknowledge my gratitude to the following colleagues at the Stanford University School of Medicine: Dr. Halsted Holman, professor of medicine, for his helpful comments and criticism; Dr. John Collins, professor of surgery, for his suggestions for modifying Chapter 9 (he agrees with much but not all of the material in that chapter); Dr. Norman Blank, professor of radiology, for valuable critical comments and suggestions on Chapters 1 through 7; Dr. James Theodore, associate professor of medicine, for help and support throughout the development of this project. He has translated into his care of patients many of the suggestions outlined in this book. Spyros Andreopoulos, director of communications for the Stanford Medical Center, offered steady encouragment and much useful criticism. I am grateful for the editorial assistance and extensive constructive criticism of an anonymous colleague. Two fourth-year medical students, Michael Lemmers and Joseph Heiserman, offered helpful criticism, and—they tell me—as a result of reading the manuscript, learned to approach patients somewhat differently. I am fortunate to have had the advice and encouragement of two Stanford residents in medicine, Dr. David Nelson and Dr. Connor Burke. The contributions of Mary Ellen Gist-Murtaugh, my friend and personal secretary, ranged from a careful personal analysis of the book to typing the manuscript.

I also acknowledge as an important source of reference, *Medicine Out of Control, The Anatomy of a Malignant Technology* (Sun Books, Melbourne, Australia, 1979) by Richard Taylor.

I disagree with many of Dr. Taylor's conclusions, but I agree with some of his material and the book has been generally helpful; in particular, a title used in his book inspired the title of Chapter 12 in my book.

Laura Ackerman-Shaw, production manager of the Portable Stanford, patiently and expertly turned the manuscript into a book. Miriam Miller, the editor of the Portable Stanford, made numerous contributions to the writing of this book. The original suggestion that the material might be of interest to the public was hers; she edited and polished the text; and, most important, she protected me—as much as one can be protected —from the inadequacies of my own writing style. I am more than grateful for her guidance.

MEDICAL CARE CAN BE DANGEROUS TO YOUR HEALTH

To protect their privacy, patients, doctors, and institutions are not identified by name or geographical location.

1

What This Book Is About

Not long ago I was involved in the care of a previously normal 40-year-old man with a family. When I examined him, he was in a deep coma. He did not respond to painful stimuli, gave no evidence of any intellectual function, and had no control of bladder or bowel. He did not move. His heart and lungs worked, his bladder and bowel functioned automatically, but there was no glimmer of specifically human behavior. He was a 40-year-old "vegetable."

I reconstructed his story from the hospital record: He had been admitted six months earlier because of fever, progressive stupor, and various neurologic abnormalities. At that time he was certainly a sick patient but definitely not a vegetable. It was thought that he might be suffering from herpes encephalitis, an infection of the brain caused by the herpes virus.

For most types of viral encephalitis, there is no specific treatment, and many patients recover spontaneously; however, herpes encephalitis is usually treated with the drug adenine arabinoside (ara-A). Although the evidence supporting its effectiveness is weak, it is the best drug available. It also has serious toxic effects; it produces severe abnormalities of the bone marrow (bone marrow manufactures various kinds of blood cells). But given the terrible prognosis of untreated herpes encephalitis—death, or irreversible brain damage—most doctors would use ara-A in a patient with definite diagnosis of herpes encephalitis.

To help resolve this dilemma—whether to use a toxic drug

in the hope of curing a terrible disease—doctors may order a brain biopsy before prescribing ara-A. Opening the skull, they remove a small amount of brain tissue, which is then examined under the microscope for signs of the herpes virus. The idea of removing any portion of the brain is, of course, awesome. In the adult, brain cells once removed are no longer replaced. Brain biopsy may be associated with irreversible and occasionally fatal complications such as bleeding into the brain.

A brain biopsy had been done on my patient. No herpes virus was found, but almost immediately following the biopsy, he sank into the coma in which I found him six months later. His condition was irreversible; he would be a vegetable for the rest of his "life."

Most of the doctors originally involved in his care were convinced that his dramatic downhill course was a result of the brain biopsy—that he had bled into the brain. It was barely possible, however, that the underlying cause was infection by the herpes virus. Brain biopsies have been known to be negative despite the presence of the virus. Therefore, even though the biopsy was negative, he was treated with ara-A. This treatment produced no improvement, and the patient and his family were condemned to a continuing horror.

The complex issues involved in this case will be analyzed more fully in Chapter 4. But the end result is clear: A patient suffered a horrible fate almost certainly as a result of a test. Doctors then ignored the outcome of the test and treated the patient as if the test had never been done. Could this disaster have been avoided? Why was the test done if the results were ultimately ignored? What went wrong?

You will learn as you read on that disasters like this one are not uncommon and that many diagnostic tests are done despite an overwhelming probability that the results will not be helpful to the patient.

No individual doctor could be blamed for the tragic outcome in my patient. Rather, the basic cause lies in a series of flaws in the system by which medical knowledge is introduced and applied to patient care—and in the way doctors are trained. These flaws foster a preoccupation with the process of diagnosis, which in this instance led to grave and irreversible damage to the patient. The outcome could not be considered the result of medical malpractice.

Malpractice consists of a breach of the community's standards of medical practice. It occurs when a physician's activities do not conform to those practiced in the community. But suppose that most of the physicians in the community are wrong about some aspect of medical care. Then this systematic error represents the standard of medical care and to conform to it is not malpractice.

This book deals largely with the nature of the systematic flaws or defects in medical care and training, rather than with the errors of individual doctors. As will become apparent, I believe that many of these flaws can be overcome by modifying the way that medical information is introduced into patient care, by modifying the way that medical information is used, and by modifying the way that doctors are trained.

I also believe that you, as a patient, can shield yourself from the consequences of many of these flaws. You face a dilemma that you may not even recognize: How to reap the benefits of modern medical care without exposing yourself to the risks. You consult doctors because the potential benefits seem obvious to you, but you are probably not aware of most of the potential risks. In fact, many doctors are not aware of them, or may underestimate their magnitude. This book will emphasize the risks chiefly because an understanding of them may help you to make better decisions with regard to your medical care.

The Risks Versus the Benefits of Reading This Book

In reading this book you stand to gain some benefits, but you also subject yourself to some risks: Your confidence in doctors could be undermined to the point where you deprive yourself of timely or even necessary medical care. That would be unfortunate. Conventional medical care does offer the best possibility of helping those who are truly sick.

You run the risk of feeling insecure in dealing with doctors. I would suggest that some measure of insecurity may be appropriate. You may learn some things that will prompt you to look back with a critical eye on your previous medical care and second-guess your current doctors—but learning from previous medical experience is useful. You may find yourself less ready to accept medical advice, but some degree of reservation is often warranted.

What are the potential benefits to you? You will gain a more realistic picture of what medicine can and cannot do for patients. This will permit you to deal more effectively with illness and with doctors. You will come to see how the medical system works. This can be intellectually satisfying but, more importantly, it can help you avoid serious errors in your own care.

You will learn, too, that some medical errors stem from the actions of patients themselves. By learning what not to do, you may increase your chances of being helped when you are ill. You will be advised to consult doctors only when you believe that you are truly ill. By restricting your medical encounters to those that are absolutely necessary, you will be avoiding the risks inherent in most diagnostic and therapeutic procedures.

This advice tends to slight an important function that doctors have assumed in our society: Dealing with patients whose main problem is an unhappy life. It is your privilege to consult a doctor for that purpose, but you should know that few doctors have high cure rates for unhappy lives, so that the chances of getting real help are small. Moreover, your visit may start a series of potentially dangerous medical tests and treatments. If, as a result of reading this book, you see that even the decision to consult a doctor is a serious and potentially risky one, that it requires some estimate of potential risks as well as potential benefits, you will have spent your time well.

You will be cautioned to avoid hospitalization unless you are seriously ill and only a hospital has the facilities for your treatment. Many hospitalizations are unnecessary and, as you will see, hospitals can be dangerous places.

Even the annual physical carries some risk, as do other kinds of routine examinations in apparently normal people, and the evidence presented here may lead you to avoid these.

You will be advised to deal with your doctor as a fellow human being and not as a god. Following this advice should improve the results of your medical care.

You will learn something about the specifics of medical knowledge in several areas of disease. This will not enable you to be your own doctor, but you will find this information intrinsically interesting as well as useful.

I believe that, on balance, the benefits of reading this book will outweigh the risks. I believe that an informed patient is an important asset in health care.

This is not an exposé of medicine. Doctor baiting is a popular sport, but not one that I care to indulge in. Most of the problems of medicine do not arise from inadequacies of individual doctors but are rooted in the medical system. To solve these problems we will have to change both medical teaching and medical care.

This volume, though not balanced in detail, is balanced in emphasis. Because the emphasis is necessarily on the potential risks of medical care, more space will be devoted to problems and less to triumphs. However, the triumphs do exist and are acknowledged.

If some of the cases I have cited as examples read like a chamber of horrors, keep in mind that they are chosen to illustrate problems, and are not necessarily typical of medical care in that area. Neither are they totally isolated instances. Each of the fifty-odd lay people and doctors who have seen parts of this book have described comparable disasters attributable to medical care.

I have deliberately refrained from giving medical advice for dealing with specific illnesses. That is not the purpose of the book. Its purpose is to reveal to you the limitations of medicine in the hope that this knowledge will help you deal more effectively with medical problems.

Many popular books tell you how to deal with individual doctors or with particular problems intrinsic to the present system of medicine. Several of these books are useful. They assume, however, that *(a)* the present system of medical care is fundamentally sound, and *(b)* the reader understands the basic workings of that system.

The present volume, by contrast, attempts to analyze the system, taking as its premise that the system rather than individual doctors is primarily responsible for the harm that patients may suffer. It assumes further that an understanding of the system and its problems will be useful to patients. The terms *medicine* and *medical system* describe the sum total of medical knowledge and medical practice generally accepted at a given time.

It has long been recognized that medicine has the potential for doing harm as well as good. What is not commonly recognized, however, is that the potential for both harm and good has increased as medical science and medical technology have progressed. The number of things that doctors can do and actually do has multiplied enormously. This growth has occurred without appropriate corresponding changes in the processes by which medical practices are established and by which doctors are trained.

I have not (with rare exception) identified specific people. This is a book without villains but with many heroes—patients who endure despite the imperfect state of medicine, and the millions of patients who have served as objects of study or experiment, thus making it possible for medicine to be as useful as it is.

Second Opinions

If reading this book troubles you, you may want to discuss it with your doctor. I have presented the material to many doctors. These are some of their reactions.

Enthusiastic support often comes from doctors who have not kept up with medicine. They see in my views a justification for their failure to keep abreast of medicine. This support makes me uneasy. My message is not anti-medical science or anti-technology. On the contrary, I personally believe that we need more, not less, science in medicine. But we need better science and a medical science more closely linked to the needs of patients. What I do criticize is the inadequate basis of medical knowledge and the common failure to recognize this inadequacy.

The very young in medicine, particularly medical students and interns, tend to be supportive. Their views have not yet hardened. Physicians who have recently completed their medical training tend to be quite negative. They read into the criticisms a challenge of the validity of what they "know" to be true. Their perception is accurate. I do challenge the validity of much of the substance of current medical practice.

Some doctors agree with the general thrust of my book but oppose carrying the message outside the family of doctors. They feel that the lay person does not have sufficient medical background or sophistication to handle the material adequately. They fear that an open public airing will lead to harm by discouraging patients from seeking needed medical care or accepting medical advice.

A number of doctors accept the validity of the criticism when leveled at other groups of doctors but reject criticism leveled at their own group. Cardiologists may be quite scornful when a gastroenterologist's mistakes are laid out. They are, however, not amused at a parallel analysis of the handling of a heart patient by one of their number. Surgeons readily accept criticism of internists but less readily accept criticism of surgeons, and so forth. Many doctors will accept the validity of some, but not all, of what is stated here. Some doctors will, of course, be convinced that this book is simply wrong and harmful to boot. I would urge you to use your own judgment.

What I Hope This Book Accomplishes

My discussion rests upon three major premises.

1. The basic processes for introducing and using diagnostic and therapeutic measures in medicine contain serious flaws.
2. Many of the flaws I describe in the body of the book can be corrected.
3. Patients can reduce the risks and increase the benefits of their medical treatment if they are aware of the flaws in our medical care system.

In writing this book I too have taken some risks but hope for some benefits. The major risk is that my criticisms may stand in the way of your getting proper medical care. I am willing to take that risk because I trust your judgment and common sense.

The major benefit to me is a sense of having provided an accurate description of the limitations of medicine in a way that improves your chances of deriving the greatest benefit from your doctor and the medical care system. That is a rich reward indeed, so I have decided to accept the risks.

2

Risk-Benefit Analysis for Patients

The principle behind risk-benefit analysis is exceedingly simple. Most decisions in life involve estimates of possible risks versus possible benefits. I decide to cross the street: The risk is that I will be hit by a car; the benefit is that I reach the other side. A formal risk-benefit analysis for this decision would, of course, be absurd; we intuitively learn to watch for cars and cross streets without thinking.

We have learned, too, that the relation between risk and benefit is altered by circumstances. Under normal circumstances, I do not try to cross a busy freeway. If, however, I see someone trapped inside a burning car on the other side of the freeway, I decide to cross. A different *benefit* has developed. I will risk being hit by a car because I may be able to save a life. My decision depends on an estimate of probability: How likely I am to be hit by a car versus how likely I am to save a life. Risk-benefit analyses usually include such an estimate of probability.

What I want to suggest here is that we need to apply the same kind of analysis to medical care, and consciously. Patients should understand that most medical care involves risks as well as benefits. Even the simple act of consulting a doctor has elements of both. When they are ill, patients tend to focus on the benefits of medical care but do not perceive the possible risks. Actually, many of the risks of medical care occur when people are well. In an annual checkup, for example, the risks are not apparent to most physicians, let alone to most patients.

9

Doctors are routinely called upon to make decisions for which they should perform risk-benefit analysis, but too often they fail to recognize the extent to which, in even simple decisions, both risk and benefit are involved.* Nor do they recognize that their decision cannot be made in an absolute sense but depends on some sort of probability estimate.

Even when a doctor knows the risks of a particular form of management, he may not transmit the information to the patient. Suppose, for example, your doctor tells you, "Do not take this medicine if you have an ulcer, ulcerlike symptoms, bleeding problems, diabetes, gout, or some forms of arthritis. Do not take it if you have asthma or are in the last three months of pregnancy. If you develop heartburn, ringing in the ears, bruises on your skin, a skin rash, wheezing, or sudden death, stop taking the medicine and get in touch with me immediately."

You would probably be alarmed at these instructions, but they are all appropriate for describing the risks of taking aspirin. Your doctor ordinarily does not give you this information. He knows that the probability of your being harmed is small and so he tells you to "cross the street." Unless you were among those few patients who develop one of the complications that aspirin causes, you would be unaware of the potential risks.

For many or most diagnostic and therapeutic procedures, the data needed for a rational decision are simply not available. Much of medical care is based on a limited and often distorted data base and limited experience, so that potential risks tend to be underestimated and potential benefits tend to be overestimated. A method does exist for rationally determining the probabilities of risk versus benefit, and that is a *clinical trial.* You will learn more about clinical trials shortly.

*There is a discipline within medical science devoted to developing methods for making risk-benefit analyses that would improve decision making by physicians. This effort is commendable, but often the data base used is so imperfect that the value of the analysis is limited. From the standpoint of patients, it is to be hoped that this discipline will flourish.

The Cost of Faulty Risk-Benefit Analysis

Let us use a *hypothetical* example to demonstrate what terrible errors can occur in medicine, how many patients may be affected by an error, and how hard it is, because of faulty risk-benefit analysis, to detect systematic errors.

Cancer of the pancreas is a difficult cancer to detect and the prognosis is poor, especially if detection comes late in the course of the disease. Let us suppose that a blood test is introduced which, when positive, is said to indicate the presence of pancreatic cancer; and when negative, to indicate no pancreatic cancer. Ten patients with known pancreatic cancer undergo the test; the test is positive in all ten. Ten controls, apparently normal subjects, believed not to have cancer of the pancreas, also undergo the test. The test is positive in one of the controls (10 percent) and negative in the other nine. (This control subject may have cancer of the pancreas; this is unlikely, but it is not possible to know with absolute certainty.) The test is repeated and the percentage of controls with positive results remains at 10 percent. These 10 percent are assumed to be false positives (cancer free), and this rate of 10 percent false positives is considered acceptable for the use of the test in the general population.

The test is accepted as a screening procedure to detect early cancer of the pancreas and thereby decrease the death rate of this killer disease. It is administered to one million subjects. Perhaps you have spotted a serious flaw. In the original study, one-half of the group had pancreatic cancer, the other half did not. In the general population, perhaps 100 patients in every million have pancreatic cancer (it is a relatively rare disease) and 999,900 do not. Therefore, the number of patients who are false positives in the general population and might come to harm by being subjected to the test is vastly greater than the number of patients with cancer of the pancreas who might benefit from early detection.

When the million subjects are tested, 50 patients with cancer of the pancreas are detected and undergo surgery. Two die of surgical complications and 20 die of complications of the cancer (surgery does not help everyone with this disease). The use of the test has saved 28 lives.

The Fate of the False Positives

But look what happens to a far larger group. Ten percent of the million subjects (100,000 *now patients*) have false-positive tests. Most of them are frightened, some to distraction. They undergo tests and surgery because they fear they may have cancer—a disease which, in fact, they almost certainly do not have. They are hospitalized and undergo extensive testing. Ten patients die during the performance of the tests. A mortality rate of one death per 10,000 tests performed is remarkably low for invasive procedures. Ultimately each of the remaining 99,990 positives undergoes surgery. Three hundred die during surgery. The test has killed 310 patients, while saving 28.

The anxiety of the surviving 99,690 false positives continues even after surgery fails to reveal any malignancy. They have been told by their surgeon that surgery does not reveal the presence of pancreatic cancer in all affected patients. Even surgical exploration produces false negatives, that is, the patient has the disease although the surgery doesn't reveal it. In other words, any of the original *false positives* may now be *false negatives*. All false positives now suffer varying degrees of chronic anxiety.

After the first year's experience, the test is evaluated by experts in the field of pancreatic cancer; they conclude that the test has resulted in an important decrease in deaths from pancreatic cancer—which it has. This news creates a big stir. The federal government and the American Cancer Society carefully monitor the death rate from various forms of cancer. The favorable results are easily detected and widely publicized.

The test has increased the death rate from unnecessary surgery, but the experts who follow deaths from surgery have nothing notable to report. Three hundred additional deaths among surgical patients is not that remarkable and, as a result, this news is not reported.

There is no agency to monitor the emotional agonies that the false-positive patients experience. There is no test to measure the degree of emotional harm inflicted on the false-positive group. Thirty-five suicides occur among them in the year of the test. But, of course, in any group of 99,690 people one must expect some suicides. These may have been unstable people to begin with. Some other "trivial" incident might have tipped them over. Whether the suicide rate is in excess of the rate expected in the general population is difficult to say. The suicides never come to public attention.

There are 15,000 divorces among the false positives in the year of the test. It is impossible to estimate whether the rate of divorce is significantly higher in this group than in the general population. The divorces are not evaluated by any experts or brought to anyone's attention. There are 1,000 bankruptcies among the false positives in the year of the test and its followup. The cost of medical care is not cheap. No one knows how many bankruptcies would have occurred in this group had they not been tested. The bankruptcies never come to public attention. Overwhelming medical consensus is that the test is of great benefit.

Suppose you had a friend in whom pancreatic cancer was detected early, and whose life may have been saved by surgery as a result of the test. Would you be inclined to doubt its benefits? If you were told that the test might cause more harm than good, would you believe that? And the doctor who administered the test to your friend—would he not feel that he had helped save a life, and could he be restrained from referring additional subjects for the test?

If you had a friend who was a false positive and died from surgery, the overwhelming chance is that you would not blame the test, since you probably would not have heard about false positives. You would mourn your friend's death but would feel that the attempt to save him from dying of cancer was justified. And would the doctor who administered the test be likely to think, "I used a test that killed a patient unnecessarily"? Hardly.

And suppose you were the patient: How would you feel about the test? If you were the patient that died, your feelings would be irrelevant.

Hidden Errors Multiply

There is more to be learned from this saga. Given the huge "success" of the screening test, efforts would be intensified to persuade people to undergo the test. "Stamp out pancreatic cancer" would become the slogan. The next year 4 million people might have the test. Now 112 lives would be saved by the test, and it would become a well-established procedure. The 400,000 people harmed would be largely overlooked.

Other benefits of the test would become apparent. If the fee for each test were set at $50, a new industry would be spawned, and by the second year would be grossing $100 million per year. Think of all the new jobs that would be created and how many people would come to depend on the blood test for their livelihood.

Consider also the fact that contributions of public money to organizations leading the fight against cancer would increase. This would permit more basic and clinical research to be performed on cancer—an obviously worthwhile result.

There are, in all likelihood, more surgeons in this country than are currently needed. The test would create new job opportunities for them. Nurses and paramedical personnel are in oversupply. They would all benefit from this new market. Our country has too many empty hospital beds; those excess beds would be filled with the false-positive patients. Almost everyone would gain except the unfortunate false-positive patients.

Admittedly, this is a hypothetical example. The results are

predicated on the figures I arbitrarily selected. If at this point you are thinking, "I did not bargain to read a work of fiction," I would urge you to withhold judgment and reread this section after you have read about cancer screening in normal subjects (Chapter 12). Whatever you decide, remember that false-positive subjects are often the hidden victims of medical testing.

The Value of Clinical Trials

Could the untoward effects of the test have been anticipated? The answer is Yes. These problems are common to most tests. Could the harm to patients have been prevented? The answer is Yes, again. A careful study of the test, performed on several thousand representative subjects before instituting its mass use, would have revealed most of its limitations, and millions of people would not have been exposed to potential risk. Called a clinical trial, this kind of limited study is a method for rationally determining the probabilities of risk versus benefit and should be mandatory. The effect of a given intervention is tested on a control group (no intervention) and an experimental group (intervention), and the results in the two groups are compared. You will learn more about clinical trials and their limitations in Chapter 8. You will also learn that harmful practices introduced into medicine tend to proliferate and become epidemic.

Clinical trials may be *prospective*—an organized study whose conditions have been pre-set by the investigator—or *retrospective*—hindsight data extracted from medical records of patients who were being managed for purposes other than the trial.

In clinical trials, foresight is considerably better than hindsight. Prospective trials are substantially more reliable than retrospective analysis. In the prospective trial the criteria for the selection of subjects can be rigorously defined. The results obtained from every patient meeting these criteria are included in the final analysis. In the prospective trial, the investigator's bias can be minimized by an appropriate experimental design. For example, the investigators gathering data may not be permitted to see individual results until the study has been completed. Whereas the data in a prospective trial is restricted to the pre-set format, in the retrospective analysis, inappropriate patients are included and the results of patients who do not fit the bias of the investigator may be excluded. The "data" for a retrospective trial have been entered into the record by a number of individuals for a variety of purposes. Even interpretation of the written record may be inaccurate.

For these and other reasons the results of retrospective clinical trials are notoriously unreliable. For example, four separate retrospective studies affirming the high accuracy of a particular test for blood clots in the lung appeared in the medical literature. When an adequate prospective trial of the accuracy of the test was performed, most of the conclusions turned out to be incorrect. The retrospective analyses were unconsciously flawed by the biases of the investigators.

Should you insist on knowing the results of an acceptable clinical trial before undergoing a test? The answer is Yes. Otherwise, you cannot assess the possible risks versus benefits, and you are denied the freedom of informed choice. Is it common practice in medicine to perform careful clinical trials before introducing tests that can affect the welfare of masses of patients? Sadly, the answer is No. This omission is one of the major systematic flaws in medicine. Incorrect medical practices do affect masses of patients. They may be difficult to detect, and may be difficult to correct once they are ingrained in medical practice. As you learn about the processes that promote systematic errors, you will more readily detect them for yourself. Raising these issues with your doctor may help both of you to become better informed.

3

What the Patient Wants or Should Want from the Doctor

A sick person wants to become healthy as completely, as rapidly, as safely, as painlessly—and perhaps as inexpensively—as possible. A healthy person wants to stay healthy. Most doctors would agree with these goals. Indeed, they can easily be transformed into a useful job description for the doctor.

A Job Description for the Doctor

In the context of a specific illness, the doctor should attempt to optimize the patient's chances for as happy and productive a life as is possible.

This statement appears simple and obvious, but it is more complex than it seems. *Attempt* is different from *succeed.* There can be no guarantee that the outcome of the doctor's attempt will be successful. Success depends on many factors, some of which are not under the doctor's control. These include the nature of the disease, the availability of effective treatment, the response of the patient to treatment, and a number of imponderables. The outcome of treatment is not the only or even the appropriate criterion by which a doctor should be judged.

The doctor may "try too hard." Overly vigorous attempts may actually reduce the chances for a happy and productive life, as they did in this instance: A male garbage collector in his thirties, married and the father of two children, had a routine chest x-ray; it was found to be grossly abnormal. He had no symptoms of disease and, indeed, had been working up until the day he entered the hospital. In the hospital, studies revealed that his primary disease was a cancer of the testicle. A biopsy of his lung performed by means of a tube introduced into his air passages showed that the cancer had spread to his lung, giving rise to the abnormal chest x-ray, and a diagnostic study of his brain revealed that the cancer had probably spread to that organ as well.

Cancer specialists were consulted. Despite the fact that the patient was without symptoms and appeared well, they decided that the cancer required emergency treatment, consisting of very large doses of various anti-cancer drugs, most of which were given by vein rather than by mouth. Within six hours of treatment, the patient deteriorated rapidly. His chest x-ray became so abnormal that no air-bearing lung tissue could be seen. Despite heroic supportive treatment, his lungs were so damaged that he was unable to obtain sufficient oxygen to survive.

It is almost certain that death was brought about by the destruction not only of cancer tissue but also of normal tissue in the lung caused by the large doses of anti-cancer drugs. This massive, rapid insult destroyed normal function of the lung, and the patient died. In retrospect, the cancer treatment was too rapid, too massive, and too vigorous; and the patient died as a result. Whether, in fact, a medical emergency existed is questionable.

Should the doctors have known in advance that the treatment was too vigorous? It is difficult to say and even experts might disagree, but the fact remains: A relatively intact young man died more quickly than necessary as a result of treatment. For the patient and his family, the result was the shortening of a happy and productive life.

When to Abandon Treatment

Doctors and public now generally agree that therapeutic efforts should be largely abandoned when brain death has occurred. There are, however, patients with problems short of brain death who are also best served by almost no treatment. To withdraw treatment is one of the most difficult decisions a physician may be called upon to make (and will be more fully discussed in Chapters 11 and 12). The general objective of treatment, as stated in our job description, is to increase the chances for a "happy and productive life." This is quite different from as long a life as possible. The difference may be illustrated by a simple equation:

$$\begin{array}{c} \text{Happy \& productive} \\ \text{life span} \end{array} = \text{life span} - \begin{array}{c} \text{Total nonhappy \&} \\ \text{nonproductive} \\ \text{life span} \end{array}$$

To assign a specific number to each term in this equation is not always possible, but the equation itself is useful in clarifying the issues involved in such a decision.

It should be understood that time spent in a hospital away from friends and family, time spent away from work, time spent in undergoing painful and undignified diagnostic and therapeutic interventions constitutes a non-happy, nonproductive life.

In many forms of cancer, for example, the efficacy of therapy is usually evaluated in terms of years of survival—five years, three years, etc. Any such evaluation may be a considerable overestimate if the criterion of happy and productive life is substituted for total life span. In one form of leukemia, acute myelogenous leukemia, a cancer of the bone marrow that attacks a specific type of white blood cell, the average life span without treatment is approximately four months. A very small number of patients may actually live for years untreated, but this happens so rarely that it cannot be considered a reasonable possibility. Chemotherapy with anti-cancer drugs prolongs the average total life span by perhaps 14 months. The treatment itself is associated with recurrent infections, fever, loss of appetite, and a series of other complications that make life miserable. During and after treatment, these patients require frequent rehospitalization. As a result, the actual prolongation of happy and productive life is considerably less than 14 months.

Because untreated patients also suffer from severe disabling symptoms, the choice between treatment and no treatment is exceptionally difficult. For the physician, the issue is not whether or not to provide the treatment—that should be the choice of the patient as guided by family and physician—but rather to make clear to the patient the problems associated with treatment so that he or she can make a reasonable choice. Most, but not all, patients would probably opt for treatment. For patients of advanced age, there is an added consideration: It may be unwise to spend much of their remaining time in a hospital undergoing complicated, dehumanizing, and painful treatment for a relatively brief prolongation of life.

To refer back to the equation, treatment may actually result in a negative quantity—it may *decrease* the length of happy and productive life. The garbage collector with cancer of the testicle and lung is a striking example.

It should be emphasized that what constitutes a happy and productive life differs from individual to individual. For some patients even a modicum of existence, however painful and uncomfortable, is precious. I once knew a patient paralyzed and confined to a rotating stretcher, but one of the most cheerful and optimistic people I have ever met. She maintained a real interest in everyone who passed through her room, and her little bit of existence was incredibly valuable. To attempt to keep her alive at almost any cost was appropriate. For other patients, even moderate degrees of confinement are intolerable, and heroic attempts to keep them alive may not be appropriate. Ideally, doctors should tailor the intensity of their efforts to the wishes of their patients.

Who Should Make the Decision?

Who should have the ultimate responsibility for defining a happy and productive life? Obviously, the patient. If the patient is unable to decide because of his condition, the patient's family should have the major voice. The doctor's role is to be friend and advisor. Because this is not always understood by patients or by physicians, patients commonly permit doctors to usurp their right to make this crucial judgment.

Consider, for example, a case recently described in a medical journal. A 58-year-old woman suffered from manic-depressive psychosis. While being treated with lithium, a drug that is effective in many patients with this disorder, she was well. But reports in the medical literature that lithium can produce permanent kidney damage worried her doctors and, as a consequence, neither her internist nor her psychiatrist was willing to continue the treatment. The drug was stopped, and she lapsed into severe mood changes that disrupted her life and the life of her family. Attempts by the patient and family to persuade the doctors to continue the drug failed. Other drugs were ineffective and the patient was thus deprived of the chance for a happy and productive life.

Her doctors were quite right, of course, to call attention to the risks of lithium, although kidney disease is a relatively rare complication of this treatment. Once informed, however, the patient had the right to decide whether the benefits for her outweighed the risks. The author of the article correctly concluded that the doctors had usurped the patient's prerogative to opt for what seemed the best choice for a happy and productive life. The doctors were not villains; they were acting in the best interests of the patient—as they saw them. But their decision was inappropriate. The possibility of permanent kidney disease represented a price to be paid for attempting to achieve what was most important to her.

This patient offers a specific example of a more general problem. Often, of course, the choices are not this clear. What should the doctor do when a patient requests a form of treatment that the doctor thinks is not indicated or is actually harmful? Suppose the patient has cancer and demands Laetrile; or is suicidal and asks for large doses of sleeping medications? Each request is a matter for the individual physician's conscience and analysis.

It is possible to understand the decision to withdraw lithium from a patient, even if it is difficult to agree with it. But how should the patient and her family have reacted? Should she have passively accepted the decision of the doctors and a miserable life along with it?

She need not, and should not, have accepted the decision to withhold lithium. If the facts were as stated, the patient almost certainly could have found a doctor who would take over her care and prescribe lithium. The doctor would share with her the responsibility for placing her at long-term risk for kidney disease but, at the same time, would be helping her reap the immediate benefits of the treatment.

Remember that, as a patient, you have the right to define the meaning of a happy and productive life for yourself. But once you exercise this right, you share the responsibilities for its consequences.

The Patient's Right to Refuse Treatment

A particularly difficult issue arises when the right of the patient to refuse treatment may result in death. Certain religious groups, for example, have decided that to receive a blood transfusion would violate their religious beliefs. When blood transfusions are required to save the patient's life, a struggle may develop between the doctor and the patient and family. That patients who are in a position to make an informed decision have the right to refuse blood transfusions is increasingly recognized. In the case of an innocent third party, such as a child, however, the doctor's opinion may be imposed and transfusions provided.*

---

*This situation has resulted in some advance for medical science. A series of blood substitutes is being tested in such patients, and the results of the tests may ultimately benefit many.

This theme—the patient's right to refuse treatment—was well portrayed in the 1970s in a play and movie, *Whose Life Is It, Anyway?* by Brian Clark. An intelligent and talented young sculptor has become completely and permanently paralyzed after an automobile accident. He has lost all voluntary body movement and is without sensation. He decides that to be an intact brain without a body is equivalent to being dead. He knows that many patients who are equally handicapped do build some kind of life for themselves, but he does not want this option for himself. He wants all treatment stopped so that his death can be completed with dignity.

He is bitterly opposed by the chief physician at the hospital. This doctor is not a bad fellow and is reasonably competent. But he is pompous, arrogant, and utterly convinced that the patient does not have the right to decide for himself that life is no longer worth living—meaning, of course, that the doctor knows best. Finally, an understanding judge decides that the patient has that right and plans are made to withhold all treatment. Presumably, the patient dies within several days.

While focusing on the right of the patient to refuse treatment, the play also highlights another interesting issue. Society has agreed to accept brain death as an indication for withholding treatment, thereby establishing the principle that life without a functioning brain is not really life. The play suggests that life with only a brain and without control of other organs is, for some patients, a form of death.

A variant of the crucial question, Who is to make the decision? arises in human heart-lung transplantation. This largely experimental procedure is being used for patients who are terminally ill with far-advanced disease of the blood vessels of the lung. To be successful, it requires the long-term use of a drug, cyclosporin-A, which has adverse effects on the kidneys and liver. Cyclosporin-A is also associated with lymphoma, a form of cancer of the lymph tissue, in a significant percentage of patients. Each candidate for heart-lung transplantation is required to decide explicitly whether to undergo a procedure which, if successful, will save his or her life in the short term and improve lifestyle quickly, or whether to forgo the procedure because of the long-term risks of cancer. What physician should feel wise enough to make the choice for the patient—cancer as the price for immediate survival? To my knowledge, every patient given this choice opts for the short-term benefit by accepting heart-lung transplant, leaving the future to take care of itself.

The present nature of the patient-physician relationship makes it difficult for many patients to express their views. Traditionally, patients have tended to be passive, a tendency aggravated by the all-too-common view of the physician as god. Typically, patients feel helpless, or at the least inadequate, before what they perceive as the infallible expertise of the doctor and are unwilling to accept the responsibility of opposing the doctor's judgment. The doctor's opinion is not infallible and you need not be passive. It is your future that is being decided. Remember that you, the patient, have the highest stake in the decision—the most to gain and the most to lose. You, the patient, if you are capable of making the decision, are the one to decide what constitutes a happy and productive life. Don't let your doctor, however well intentioned, usurp this right.

Diagnostic Efficiency Versus Therapeutic Efficiency

Some elements of patient management that seem important to physicians are excluded from the job description I suggest, because these elements may be tangential to providing the best opportunity for a happy and productive life, or may even detract from that possibility. These include diagnosis, the use of patients for the doctor's education, and the use of patients for medical research.

Consider diagnosis. An 87-year-old man was relatively hale

and hearty and led an active and highly satisfactory life. He developed pain in the legs during exercise—intermittent claudication—caused by decreased blood supply to the muscles of the legs. This symptom was annoying and to some degree interfered with his usual activities. He consulted a doctor and was admitted to a hospital. One of the causes of intermittent claudication is a diseased aorta, the major arterial blood vessel from which all other arteries arise as branches to supply blood to the various organs in the body. It was therefore decided to perform an aortogram, a diagnostic procedure in which an injection of radiopaque material into a segment of the aorta is followed by x-rays of portions of the aorta that might be diseased. The purpose of this invasive test was to determine whether surgery on a potentially diseased part of the aorta might be performed to relieve the symptoms. The radiopaque material was injected through a catheter inserted into the lower part of the aorta, which supplies blood to the legs.

The doctors then decided to use the same catheter to investigate the internal carotid arteries, which supply blood to the brain. The patient had no symptoms to suggest that the blood vessels of his brain were diseased, nor would he have been a candidate for surgery of the internal carotid arteries even if disease had been found—given his lack of symptoms and his advanced age. Radiopaque material was injected directly into both carotid arteries, as a result of which he suffered a major stroke. Converted into a vegetable without thought, response, or movement, he is doomed to spend the rest of his life being fed through a tube—speechless, paralyzed, incontinent, and a burden to his family.

This patient was not a victim of bad luck. He was a victim of bad judgment fostered by a medical system that emphasizes diagnosis as an end unto itself, divorced from treatment.

Is this terrible case an example of medical malpractice on the part of his doctors? Probably not. Malpractice occurs only when the medical standards of the community are violated.

The performance of the unnecessary and ill-advised test varies from common practice only in its disastrous results.

Our job description for doctors says nothing about diagnosis, although diagnostic efforts frequently dominate medical care. It is intuitively obvious, however, that diagnostic efforts are useful to patients only as they serve to maximize the chances for a happy and productive life. Too few doctors understand the difference between diagnostic efficiency and therapeutic efficiency. A test may have high diagnostic efficiency but low therapeutic efficiency.

The difference between diagnostic efficiency and therapeutic efficiency is critical. Tests should have high therapeutic efficiency; diagnostic efficiency alone is not helpful to the patient. Finding out what is wrong is not helpful if the doctor cannot use the information to treat the patient more effectively. Consider, for example, an 83-year-old woman with

---

Diagnostic efficiency provides an index of the effectiveness of a given test by relating the number of times a given procedure results in a diagnosis to the total number of times the procedure is performed. It can be stated in a simple equation.

$$\frac{\text{Diagnostic}}{\text{efficiency}} = \frac{\text{Number of diagnoses resulting from procedure}}{\text{Total number of procedures}}$$

Therapeutic efficiency provides an index of the effectiveness of a given test in indicating proper therapy by relating the number of times effective management results from a given test to the total number of times the procedure is performed.

$$\frac{\text{Therapeutic}}{\text{efficiency}} = \frac{\text{Number of effective therapeutic decisions}}{\text{Total number of procedures}}$$

known metastatic cancer of the breast, who developed massive bleeding from her gastrointestinal tract and was admitted to a hospital. The patient, her primary physician, and her family all agreed that no surgery would be performed to treat her gastrointestinal bleeding. She would be managed conservatively with blood transfusions and drugs administered for the purpose of controlling the bleeding.

Despite the decision not to operate, she was subjected to upper gastrointestinal (GI) endoscopy. A fiberoptic tube was passed into the esophagus, stomach, and duodenum and used to detect possible sites of gastrointestinal bleeding. The primary purpose of upper GI endoscopy is to identify sites of bleeding should surgery be required. This test has its own inherent morbidity and a very small mortality. In the patient for whom a decision had been made not to operate because of her age, her cancer, and other factors, it is difficult to justify the procedure.

Her doctors should have analyzed her problem as follows:

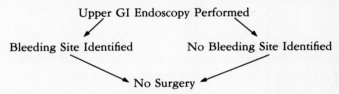

Whatever the outcome of the test, the management of the patient would be the same. The likelihood that this procedure would benefit the patient was slight.

Nor was there statistical support for the decision to perform an endoscopy. On the contrary, a series of studies reported from various medical centers show that upper GI endoscopy improves *diagnostic efficiency,* but does not improve *therapeutic efficiency* in patients with upper gastrointestinal bleeding. Whether they undergo the test or not, these patients statistically spend the same amount of time in the hospital, require the same number of transfusions, and die at the same rate; several years after the bleeding episode, their status is no different. Although there are some specific circumstances in which this procedure is indicated, it should not be routinely done on patients with upper GI bleeding.

Why then was it done on an 83-year-old cancer patient? Almost certainly because it is customary to subject patients with upper GI bleeding to the test despite the fact that, to the best of our knowledge, it will not help them. The difference between diagnostic efficiency and therapeutic efficiency is blurred in most physicians' minds.

One of the most alarming aspects of modern medicine is that, for most procedures, we know neither the diagnostic efficiency nor the therapeutic efficiency. Huge numbers of diagnostic studies, many of them invasive, are introduced into medicine, each with some morbidity and mortality, often without a general evaluation of their usefulness and often without an analysis of their role in the management of a specific patient. We will return to this problem in Chapter 4.

Educating the Doctor

The job description we established at the beginning of this chapter deliberately excludes the goal of educating the doctor. Let us examine that complicated subject. Society appears to have sanctioned the use of patients to further the education of physicians. Early in their training, when they are still quite inexperienced, medical students are given responsibilities for patient management. They usually, but not always, are closely supervised, and the practice may work out quite well for the patient. Students often make up for lack of experience by their enthusiasm, high motivation, and intensity of effort. Learning by managing patients is essential to a doctor's training, and, at the least, is in the best interests of society. It is difficult to see how this might be changed.

A variant of this theme occurs annually. There is an undocumented but strong impression among experienced physicians that July and August of each year are particularly bad months to be hospitalized in the United States. In July, newly graduated interns and residents take over major care responsibilities in most hospitals. In addition to the problems created by their inexperience, the complete change of staff makes for a substantial amount of disorganization for several weeks. But postgraduate training and clinical experience are indispensable to the training of competent doctors and therefore the practice is sanctioned. Newly trained physicians not uncommonly function better than their more experienced colleagues. Moreover, the minute-to-minute coverage of patients is better in hospitals with interns and residents than in those without house staff. Perhaps the influx of new physicians could be arranged to avoid a complete change of staff, but the outcome of the practice for society is beneficial and individual patients generally accept the idea. (An occasional patient does request "a real doctor, not an intern," and many patients choose to stay away from hospitals with interns and residents. The ratio of risks to benefits of this choice is not clear.)

Now we come to a less defensible practice. A newly devised invasive procedure is introduced into medical practice, and the group introducing it goes through a learning process. The morbidity and mortality of the procedure, as might be expected, tend to be highest at the time of introduction and to decrease as the group accumulates experience. Now the procedure becomes widely adopted and is made available at many hospitals. Each new hospital goes through the same learning process, with consequent high morbidity and high mortality. Patients managed early in the learning phase are sacrificed because of relative inexperience. That the sacrifice is not an inevitable consequence of their disease is usually not apparent to the patient or the patient's family.

Some centers never catch up. The high death rates for heart surgery in some medical centers are scandalous. A number of institutions have had, or continue to have, death rates not only far in excess of those of the best centers, but also far above the national average. Little has been done to resolve this problem. One solution would be to limit the spread of potentially risky new procedures to specific centers, so that patients would be managed at relatively experienced hospitals. The current lack of control makes for a wide range of competency and reaps an inevitable toll.

Not all doctors are equally competent, not all hospitals provide the same level of care, and not all medical centers are equally well equipped and organized. As a patient, you have the right to expect the best that medicine has to offer. Unless you ask and insist, you may settle for less than the best.

What is the response of doctors to the privilege of learning by using patients? It is a feeling, usually unformulated and unrecognized, that learning at the patient's expense is an intrinsic right of the physician, rather than a privilege granted by patients and society. Doctors often feel free to study a patient as an intellectual exercise, even though the predictable benefit for the patient is remote. Questioned about a given test, the doctor not uncommonly states that the results are "of interest"—to whom is not made clear, usually to the doctor. Often the doctor will say, "I ordered the test to make me feel more comfortable." The purpose of medical care should be to make the patient, not the doctor, feel more comfortable.

Most patients do not mind improving the education of the doctor as long as it does not threaten their own well-being. As a patient, you have the right to determine why a given series of studies and procedures is done.

Advancing Medical Science

Our job description also excludes the use of the patient to advance medical science. The advancement of medical science is a laudable goal, but it can also interfere with helping the patient. You will read more about this in Chapter 13. Undisciplined, desultory studies conducted by individual doctors usually do not advance medical science significantly nor do they usually help patients. Most patients do not mind advancing medical science unless it is at the expense of their well-being. But here again, you have the right not to be used to advance medical science.

Finally, do not conclude that doctors deliberately and with malice aforethought set out to do tangential diagnostic studies or to use patients as teaching aids or as guinea pigs. Such practices are part of the system. This being the case, it should be our goal to change the system. As a patient, insist that your doctor have your happiness and productivity as the *explicit* objective of his management. If in doubt about any test, have him explain.

The issues we have discussed in this chapter are both important and complex. They are worth reemphasizing: You and your doctor have a common goal—that you get well as quickly and as safely as possible and stay well. However, much of what the doctor does may be tangential or even contrary to this goal. Too aggressive treatment can cause harm or death. You must be the final judge of what, for you, constitutes a more happy and productive life. This may lead you to insist on therapy that the doctor feels is dangerous; or to decline therapy that, to him, seems essential. Assuming that you understand the issues, the choice should be yours, but it should be an informed choice.

Tests are useful only if they serve directly to improve your chances for a more happy and productive life. This is often not the case. Your care should not have the goal of educating the doctor. You may be willing to help educate him, but not by putting yourself at risk. Nor should your care be geared to advancing medical science unless you explicitly decide that you want to do so.

4

How Doctors Manage Illness

Management, or *clinical management,* refers to the sum total of the diagnostic and therapeutic efforts that a doctor undertakes on the patient's behalf. By tradition, training, habit, and experience, doctors usually assume that their management of individual patients reflects a favorable risk-benefit analysis. This may or may not be true.

The Workup

Patient management begins with a workup: The taking of a history, a physical examination, some general laboratory tests, and some specific procedures. First the doctor asks the patient to state his chief complaint—the immediate problem that has brought the patient to the doctor's office. (Please don't answer, "You're the doctor, you tell me." The more precise and clear your answers, the more help the doctor can ultimately provide.)

The doctor then asks the patient to describe the development of the present illness. As he listens, the doctor attempts to understand the evolution of the disease, to identify the organs that may be involved, and to gather details that may provide clues to a correct diagnosis. The doctor actively prompts the patient during the questioning, hoping to elicit a familiar pattern that will assist him in making a diagnosis.

The Medical History

A medical history—previous illnesses, medications, hospitalizations, surgery—helps the doctor gain an overall impression of the health status of the patient, as well as clues to the present illness. The doctor may also pursue a family medical history. Many diseases have, or seem to have, a hereditary basis (bronchial asthma, for example); others may depend on family contacts (infections like tuberculosis).

Next comes a review of systems, a series of questions that may start with the patient's head and end with the extremities: Headaches, fainting spells, problems with eyes, difficulties with ears, nose and throat symptoms, symptoms of chest disease, symptoms of heart disease, abdominal symptoms, symptoms involving the extremities, and signs of nervous system disease.

The patient's answers are necessarily subjective and may suggest false leads. Much of what the doctor hears is nonspecific: A complaint of fatigue calls up vast possibilities, ranging from a disease of the adrenal glands (which afflicts perhaps one in many thousands) to boredom (very common). But some information is very specific: If you have coughed up blood, this suggests to the doctor the overwhelming probability that you have a disease of the respiratory tract.

Under some circumstances, the history is short-circuited. A victim of an automobile accident may be asked few or no questions except, perhaps, how he plans to pay for his health care. On the whole, the medical history is one of the most useful approaches to diagnosing and managing individual patients. It provides not only clues to special medical problems, but also an opportunity to size up the patient as a human being. The patient should also use the occasion to size up the doctor as a human being. Despite its value, a medical history often has low sensitivity (diseases are overlooked), low specificity (diseases that are not present are suspected), and low accuracy.

The Physical Examination

A physical examination usually follows the history. The doctor uses his eyes, ears, hands, and a few simple instruments to elicit data. A detailed survey of the patient's physical status begins with the measurement of the so-called vital signs— temperature, pulse, blood pressure, and rate of breathing. Next, the doctor, starting at the patient's head, systematically examines the various organ systems, whether or not he thinks disease is present. The physical examination may or may not provide pertinent information about the patient's immediate complaint. Some findings are nonspecific: "The patient is unusually pale." Pallor may be normal for the particular patient, or may be caused by a profound anemia. But the data may be quite specific: "The patient has a particular kind of heart murmur"; the doctor may be certain that the patient has a disease of a specific heart valve.

The physical examination is frequently abbreviated—no one expects eye doctors to perform heart examinations. It may also be abbreviated in order to focus on the organ that appears to be diseased, or sometimes because of time pressures or simple lack of interest.

Medical schools inculcate in doctors-to-be the importance of performing a complete physical examination. A number of aphorisms are offered to support this practice; every student is taught, "Always perform a rectal examination, because if you don't put your finger in it, you may put your foot in it." But the largely subjective nature of much of the data acquired in the physical examination is seldom stressed. For example, medical textbooks usually define the normal rate of breathing in an adult as 16 to 20 breaths per minute. The more accurate figure is 8 to 12 breaths per minute. Because doctors and nurses are influenced by the textbooks, most medical records, not surprisingly, list the patient as having approximately 20 breaths per minute. The observer records what he considers to be accurate rather than the actual rate of breathing.

THE LIMITATIONS OF PHYSICAL EXAMINATION. False-negative and false-positive findings during physical examinations are common. A false negative overlooks a finding that is actually present, so that a disease that may be treatable is not diagnosed. In the following instance, failure to recognize a physical finding was disastrous: A 44-year-old male, alcoholic and with liver disease, became semi-stuporous. During the initial physical examination, it was not recognized that the patient had a stiff neck (less likely, the stiff neck may not have been present during the initial examination). A stiff neck suggests the possibility of meningitis, an infection of the membranes covering the brain, and would ordinarily prompt the doctor to perform an examination of the spinal fluid. Many forms of meningitis are curable by treatment with antibiotics, but because the stiff neck was not detected, the patient was treated only for the liver disease assumed to be the cause of his stupor. About six hours later, another doctor found that the patient had a stiff neck. A spinal fluid examination showed the presence of a form of meningitis. Caused by bacteria, it can be treated with specific antibiotics, but early treatment is imperative. The patient was treated, but died. The six-hour delay in treatment may have made the difference between life and death.

In a false-positive finding the doctor believes that he has identified a manifestation that in actuality does not exist. As a result, patient management is based on a spurious finding. A normal 54-year-old woman undergoes a complete physical as part of an annual health examination. During the examination of the belly, the doctor thinks he feels a large mass that could be cancer. He subjects the patient to an extensive series of tests which fail to reveal any abnormalities.

Until the results are available, the patient suffers severe anxiety.

Physicians frequently do not recognize that their inaccuracies may lead to management decisions that can harm their patients. Most physicians are unaware of the rate of either false positives or false negatives in their own use of the physical examination; nor is the statistical rate for the profession as a whole usually known.

Study reveals that physical examination is subject to great observer error, leading to high rates of false positives and false negatives. The following is an example: Cyanosis is a bluish discoloration of the skin and lips which can be produced by having normal subjects breathe mixtures low in oxygen. A panel of distinguished experts in physical diagnosis was assembled as subjects breathed various gas mixtures. Some mixtures were low in oxygen and thus caused cyanosis; others contained normal amounts of oxygen and were not associated with cyanosis. None of the doctors accurately identified when the subjects were cyanotic and when they were not. Similar studies of the accuracy of physical examination in evaluating the accuracy of other findings have produced comparable results. Physical examination is nevertheless a useful and convenient approach to diagnosis; it is largely noninvasive and therefore safe.

Routine Tests

Some general nonspecific laboratory tests are included in the workup—usually a blood count, a urinalysis, some chemical measurements of the blood; not uncommonly, a chest x-ray; and quite commonly, an electrocardiogram. The nature of these tests and their number are established by tradition, by general usage, and by convenience. Their value for most patients has not been established. There is also an economic incentive at work—it is customary to overcharge for laboratory work. Data on the effectiveness of nonspecific laboratory studies in patient care, however, are scant. What is more important, individual doctors, not knowing the risks versus benefits, often order them routinely.

If you have been a patient, you have observed that you are subjected to many tests. In fact, you may equate the intensity of testing with the excellence of the doctor—the greater their number and the more complex the studies, the better the doctor. You can be sure that many of these studies will not benefit you and some may indeed harm you. Some overtesting is inevitable, but much could be avoided if your doctor were trained differently or learned to practice differently.

Diagnostic Studies

The workup concludes with a series of specialized studies designed to result in a specific diagnosis. In selecting the specialized studies that complete the workup, the doctor is guided by the history, the physical examination, and the general laboratory tests. As science and technology have progressed, the number and range of special studies has increased and the studies have become more invasive. Much of modern medicine consists in selecting the "proper" tests from what has become a bewildering array.

Too little effort has been made to validate the usefulness of many of the studies; often their theoretical basis as well as their limitations are poorly understood by the doctor ordering them. A physician may order a test, discover that the result is abnormal, and then question the laboratories as to the meaning of the abnormality.

Having conducted a workup, the doctor expects to make a diagnosis or diagnoses; this will enable him, he believes, to develop a plan for treating the patient rationally.

Clinical Management Model

What has been described is the model that most doctors implicitly use in managing illness (see Figure 4-1).

You will note that the doctors' model rests on two assump-

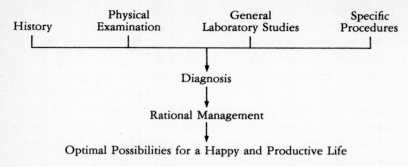

Figure 4-1. The usual model for managing illness.

tions: That diagnosis and treatment are closely linked and that treatment and a happy and productive life are also coupled. Given these assumptions, it is not surprising that diagnostic efforts are emphasized almost as an end in themselves by many doctors. While intellectually appealing, however, these assumptions prove to be incorrect. Diagnostic measures are not invariably accurate or safe, and there is not an effective form of treatment for each diagnosis.

Consider this example. A 74-year-old woman developed an illness characterized by fever, weakness, and fatigue; her chest x-ray showed many infiltrates (abnormal shadows) in the lung. When noninvasive studies failed to reveal the cause of her symptoms, an open-lung biopsy was scheduled. This meant that her chest would be opened and a piece of lung tissue removed and studied in an attempt to make a diagnosis. True, only a very few patients die of this procedure; but it is painful, produces substantial discomfort, and results in abnormalities of lung function at least temporarily. It is hardly a procedure you would recommend for your grandmother.

It was noted—before the biopsy could be performed—that the patient had begun to improve spontaneously. Her fever decreased, she felt better, and her chest x-ray became more nearly normal. Despite her obvious improvement, the lung biopsy was not postponed but was carried out as scheduled. It did reveal the presence of an infection, but one for which there is no satisfactory treatment—cytomegalovirus infection; spontaneous recovery is the rule. And, indeed, despite the surgery, this 74-year-old patient continued to recover.

The patient was presented at a teaching conference of a famous hospital as an example of the value of performing lung biopsies. The value was that the biopsy resulted in a definite diagnosis. However, it was not made clear who benefited from the test—it was certainly not the patient.

Whether this patient should ever have been scheduled for a lung biopsy is perhaps debatable. To have performed the operation when she was improving is almost inconceivable. After all, operations are not like Broadway plays; the show does not have to go on! To use the example of this patient as a general justification for performing lung biopsies is a mockery of patient care. The final irony was that the biopsy proved to be useless from the standpoint of guiding treatment for the patient, as there is no specific treatment available for her disease.

A more complex example: A 44-year-old male with heart disease entered a hospital. It became apparent that his disease was a manifestation of one of three abnormalities: Pericarditis, a disorder of the pericardium—the membrane covering the heart—for which the treatment would be surgical removal of the pericardium; myocarditis, a disorder of the heart muscle, for which no satisfactory specific treatment exists; or a simultaneous involvement of both the pericardium and the myocardium. In the latter instance, the pericardium is surgically removed and the patient is left with myocardial disease. Even when pericarditis is only a remote possibility, surgery is usually performed, because this particular disease responds well to surgical treatment. Treatment of myocarditis, on the other hand, is usually unsatisfactory.

To distinguish among these three possibilities—pericarditis, myocarditis, or both—is difficult without surgery. Surgery was therefore indicated and agreed upon. The patient was nevertheless first subjected to a series of tests, some of which are invasive and can cause morbidity or even death, in an attempt to determine the more probable diagnosis—pericardial or myocardial disease. Fortunately, the test results were largely ignored—they favored, if anything, myocardial disease. Surgery was performed and pericardial disease identified.

One would be hard put to justify exposing the patient to the risk of multiple tests that would not alter the obviously correct decision: To perform surgery in order to determine the specific disorder. Again, the value of these studies was not to the patient.

A third and final example: A 68-year-old male, bedridden and disoriented in time and space, suffered from alcoholism and dementia. He could not function adequately, except at home and under close supervision. The dementia was chronic, severe, and disabling, although its exact cause was not clear. He also had an abnormal heart valve.

In the hospital he underwent cardiac catheterization—a tube was passed into the right side of his heart and another into the left side—so that measurements could be made to determine whether he required surgical correction of the heart valve abnormality. This procedure has a low but significant associated morbidity and mortality. But only after catheterization did his doctors consider whether cardiac surgery was appropriate for this particular patient. His age and severe mental disturbances, they decided, made surgery inadvisable. They could and should have made this decision before the invasive study was performed. Catheterization was not only unnecessary but inadvisable.

The management of all three of these patients is characterized by the performance of specific diagnostic studies that were *predictably* of little or no benefit to the patient. These are isolated examples of mismanagement, but in each the incorrect decision is attributable to the same underlying systematic cause—the misplaced emphasis on diagnostic procedures—that pervades modern medicine.

The Value of Brain Biopsy

The systematic nature of the error we have been discussing —the misplaced emphasis on diagnosis—is most dramatically illustrated by the misuse of brain biopsy.

In a brain biopsy, you will recall from Chapter 1, the patient's skull is opened and a part of the brain is removed for study. If the thought of submitting to this gives you pause, you are not alone—it does most people. The brain is properly regarded as the major organ that determines our attributes as humans. Once removed, the cells of the brain do not replace themselves.

Alzheimer's Disease

The first example has to do with Alzheimer's disease, a disease of the brain common in aging patients. Characterized by progressive dementia (loss of intellectual functions over time), it is by far the most common cause of senile dementia, said to be the fourth leading cause of death in the United States (heart disease is first; cancer, second; and stroke, third). It has been known to run in families, but only rarely; the inherited form is so uncommon that it can be ignored as a possibility.

Brain tissue of persons afflicted with Alzheimer's disease, examined under the microscope, reveals more or less characteristic findings. No satisfactory treatment exists, however, so that to establish the diagnosis is essentially useless for the patient and the patient's family. But, as we have seen, there is a strong feeling that "the show must go on, the diagnostic procedure must be performed." Here is a passage from a recent editorial in a prominent medical journal:

> The clinician may easily succumb to diagnostic nihilism, discouraged by the need for a brain biopsy to delineate the precise form of presenile dementia [Alzheimer's disease]. . . . Accurate diagnosis is essential to determine the prognosis and to advise

close relatives who are worried about their risk of becoming demented in the future.

Let us translate these words into easily understandable English: A doctor who does not believe that diagnosis for its own sake is an acceptable part of patient care is a "diagnostic nihilist." The editorial writer evidently believes that, independent of its usefulness to the patient, establishing a diagnosis serves a worthwhile purpose. For Alzheimer's disease, a firm diagnosis that will help the doctor to predict its outcome and to advise relatives about their possible risks can be made only by a brain biopsy. His conclusion, therefore, is that brain biopsies should be performed on patients with suspected Alzheimer's disease.

The supposed benefit of brain biopsy in Alzheimer's disease is to achieve a diagnosis of a disease for which there is no satisfactory treatment. Will close relatives of the patient benefit? No. Even if the patient had Alzheimer's, it is most unlikely that the relatives would develop the disease. They would only be subjected to needless worries for the rest of their lives. Is the diagnosis useful for genetic counseling? Not when the patient is 60 years of age or older and the patient's relatives have already raised families. The most that could be accomplished would be to transfer severe (usually unfounded) anxieties to future generations of the unfortunate family.

In fairness, we can state that it is improbable that brain biopsy is commonly done in Alzheimer's; however, advocacy of brain biopsy demonstrates the degree to which medical diagnosis may be pushed.

Herpes Encephalitis

To return to a more particular example: You may recall the 40-year-old man, presented in Chapter 1, hopelessly disabled by overwhelming brain damage after a brain biopsy. The biopsy was performed to establish a diagnosis of herpes encephalitis, a dreaded form of virus infection of the brain with a high mortality.

The drug used for treating this disease—adenine arabinoside (ara-A) is potentially toxic and subjects patients to the hazards of excess fluid administration and damage to the bone marrow. Since the untreated disease is frequently fatal, however, most doctors treat patients with an established diagnosis of herpes encephalitis with ara-A. Some doctors believe that a tissue diagnosis of herpes encephalitis should be made before subjecting the patient to this dangerous form of therapy. A tissue diagnosis can be made only by means of a brain biopsy.

On the other hand, doctors will usually treat suspected herpes encephalitis with ara-A even when the brain biopsy is negative. This is not illogical in itself, as false-negative brain biopsies do occur. (A quoted figure for the false-negative rate is 4 percent, but there is reason to believe that it is substantially higher.) For our patient, the brain biopsy was negative for herpes encephalitis, but he was still treated with ara-A—which produced no improvement. Given the fact that doctors will use ara-A whether the brain biopsy is positive or negative, it is difficult to justify performing the biopsy. It does not influence treatment: If the brain biopsy is positive, the patient is treated with ara-A; if the brain biopsy is negative, the patient is treated with ara-A; if the brain biopsy is indeterminate, the patient is treated with ara-A. Not many experts have realized the anomaly of this common practice.

This approach is strikingly inconsistent (see Figure 4-2). Suppose a patient is treated with ara-A without a brain biopsy. The rationale would be an empirical trial of a potentially helpful drug in a desperately ill patient. This would be unacceptable, because it is contrary to the advice of the experts in the field. If the patient developed severe bone marrow toxicity, perhaps even died of ara-A administration, his doctors would be strongly criticized. One might even imagine a malpractice suit.

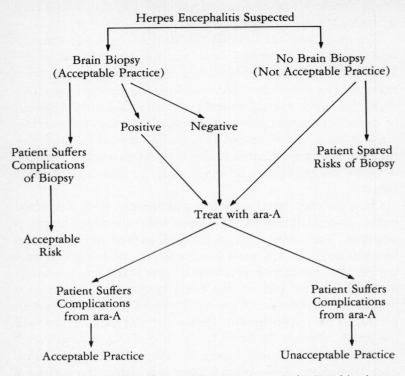

Figure 4-2. The evaluation of the patient's management is dominated by the test rather than the outcome for the patient.

But if the brain biopsy is performed and is *negative,* an empirical trial with ara-A can be justified in the eyes of experts. False-negative biopsies do occur in patients with herpes encephalitis. If now the patient develops a toxic reaction to ara-A, the doctor would not be subject to criticism. Thus, the act of performing a brain biopsy justifies a course of management no different from that which would be pursued had no brain biopsy been performed. A diagnostic test, whether helpful or not, becomes the dominant factor in patient management. This is a perversion of the goal of optimizing the patient's chances for a more happy and productive life.

Creutzfeldt-Jakob Disease

Brain biopsies were formerly performed in Creutzfeldt-Jakob disease, a devastating brain disease found in middle-aged and older adults. It produces abnormalities of behavior, emotions, memory, reasoning, hearing, and vision. The patients also develop myloclonus, peculiar jerking movements of their muscles. The disease progresses with such great rapidity that deterioration may be seen from day to day. There is no satisfactory treatment; patients with Creutzfeldt-Jakob disease usually die within one year of the onset of the disease.

There is substantial evidence that the disease is produced by a virus. Two neurosurgeons who performed brain biopsies on patients with this illness developed the disease and died. It was concluded that they acquired the disease while performing a biopsy, so biopsy is now considered too dangerous to the doctors performing the test and it has been largely abandoned. If brain biopsies had been vital to the welfare of affected patients, it is probable that doctors would have continued to perform them even at the risk of their own lives. It may, therefore, be inferred that brain biopsies were never vital to the welfare of these patients and should never have been performed.

Who Benefits from Brain Biopsies?

If you have a relative with Alzheimer's or herpes encephalitis or other brain disease, you may be informed that brain biopsy could be of value to other patients similarly affected even if not to your relative; that the best hope for finding a cure is to learn more about the given disease; and that by agreeing to a brain biopsy on your relative you will further this goal. (The patient usually is not in a position to make a decision.) In view of the slight possibility that the disease could be hereditary, you may be told that the results might be helpful to members of your family, present and future.

Do not be misled. The implicit agreement between patient and physician does not bind the patient to contribute either to medical science or to future generations. The doctor's job is to attempt to improve the well-being of the patient. The doctor has no right to demand more.

How much truth is there in the claim that brain biopsy can advance medical science? Perhaps a little, although the increment in knowledge is probably trivial. Important advances in knowledge will have to come from other approaches.

I will complete the subject of brain biopsy with an example that readers should evaluate for themselves. A group of psychotic youngsters in a child psychiatry unit—not in the United States—were subjected to brain biopsies for investigative purposes. The doctors in charge of this project concluded that even though the studies had no therapeutic consequences for the patients, they would contribute to a better understanding of the prognosis and therefore to a future improvement or understanding of the patient's problem. "It must be concluded," they reported, "that future research on the unknown etiological conditions of these serious psychic ailments should continue with brain biopsies; however, not as routine examinations, but only after consultation with all special departments involved."

We may conclude that with rare exception the performance of brain biopsies stems from diagnostic zeal and makes little or no contribution to patient welfare. Brain biopsy in most circumstances is therefore an example of a systematic error in medical management.*

A Realistic Model for Clinical Management

Let us now look at a model of patient management (see Figure 4-3) that conforms more closely to reality than does the

---

*Brain biopsy while performing surgery to remove a brain tumor usually does not increase the risk and may provide information that is useful in treatment.

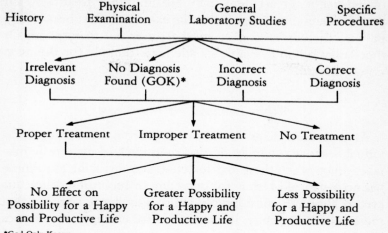

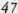

Figure 4-3. Flow diagram of the possible outcomes of a medical workup. Note that all of the possible diagnostic outcomes may have the same effect on the appropriateness of the treatment, and any treatment—proper, improper, or no treatment—may have the same effect on the ultimate outcome. The doctor's task is to determine the diagnostic and therapeutic approach that will most probably lead to a happy outcome. In life, diagnosis and management are not always very closely linked; nor are management and a happy outcome.

model presented earlier. It is more complex than the model most doctors believe in, and the experienced doctor recognizes that it is much more accurate.

Following the workup, the doctor may indeed arrive at an accurate diagnosis that will enable him to prescribe an effective treatment: A patient consults a doctor because of fever, chest pain, and bloody sputum; physical examination and chest x-ray indicate that the patient has pneumonia; the laboratory examines the sputum and finds germs known to be a common cause of pneumonia; the patient is treated with penicillin and recovers. One could argue that penicillin could have been prescribed without identifying the germ and the same result would have been achieved, but that argument is contentious.

Of course, there is always the possibility that, despite a correct diagnosis, the doctor, through lack of knowledge, lack of judgment, or accident, may use improper treatment. Or proper treatment may not have the expected effect because the patient, for one reason or another, may fail to respond. Or there may be no available or adequate remedy for the diagnosed disease.

When Diagnosis Is Inaccurate

An inaccurate diagnosis may emerge from the workup. Individual doctors generally do not keep track of diagnostic mistakes, even when these are detected, and medicine as a whole has no organized system for detecting or recording diagnostic errors, although considerable indirect evidence suggests that these occur frequently. It is no secret, for example, that masses of doctors have diagnosed diseases that never existed. *Status thymaticus* was a popular disorder in the 1920s, supposedly affecting young children and caused by a hypothetical overgrowth of the thymus gland which was frequently treated by x-ray to the neck. Not only was there no such disease, but the treatment gave rise to an increased incidence of cancer of the thyroid in these children in later years.

The emotional consequences of misdiagnosis can be severe. Here is a particularly devastating example: A young woman physician had an ultrasound test to investigate bleeding from the vagina in the first trimester of pregnancy. In an ultrasound test sound waves are used to outline various body structures —in this case, the baby. Seeing no movement in the baby, the examining doctor—a specialist in ultrasonography—concluded that the baby was dead. During the next weeks, the woman mourned the loss of her baby but refused to undergo curettage to get rid of the dead baby.

Some weeks later, during a follow-up ultrasound test, the baby did a "somersault"—it was alive! The remainder of her pregnancy was marked by severe emotional stress: Which of the two diagnoses should she trust—was her baby dead or alive?

That an ultrasound test was necessary at all is doubtful. A

more acceptable course might have been to wait and see whether the bleeding would stop. In spite of its inaccuracies, the routine use of ultrasound tests on all or most pregnant women has been advocated by some specialists.

To reiterate—*every* test has the potential to cause harm; every test has its own inherent risks. An unnecessary test, by definition, has no benefit, and the risk-benefit ratio is obviously unacceptable to the patient. When false diagnosis leads to inappropriate treatment, the patient may improve spontaneously despite the treatment; may be unaffected by the treatment; or may be harmed, or even die, as a result of the treatment.

GOK (God Only Knows)

Often diagnostic studies elicit the diagnosis GOK (God Only Knows). The failure to make a diagnosis in hospitalized patients is much more common than most physicians recognize. A survey of 200 patients admitted without diagnosis— 100 at each of two hospitals, one a university hospital and one a community hospital—disclosed that approximately 35 percent of the patients at each institution were discharged without a specific diagnosis.

GOK in some instances stems from the fact that the pathologist, who is considered the diagnostic court of final appeal, may not be able to make a definite diagnosis. Even after a biopsy and careful microscopic examination of tissue by specialized diagnostic methods, the final verdict may still be GOK.

One would expect the percentage of patients with GOK to be a function of how intensively diagnostic measures are pursued—the more intensive the effort, the less frequent the GOKs. But the fact is that, in current practice, even with aggressive pursuit of diagnosis, many disorders are simply not diagnosable. Given a diagnosis of GOK, however, the patient must still be, and is, treated, with varying results.

A final possibility is that a diagnosis irrelevant to the patient's immediate problem may emerge. This can be helpful, harmful, or have no effect.

Therapeutic Outcomes

Treatment may optimize the chances for a happy and productive life. This is, of course, what the patient wants from the doctor.

Treatment may harm the patient. This possibility is present with almost every form of treatment and is a major reason why medicine is potentially dangerous to your health. Under some circumstances, the harm is unavoidable and the risks are necessary. Under others, the risks are either avoidable or can be minimized.

The patient may recover independently of the treatment. In fact, most illnesses physicians treat successfully are self-limited and spontaneously cure themselves. Were this not true, the medical record of doctors would be grim indeed. When patients do well, doctors tend to take credit whether or not their role was significant in the outcome. When patients do badly, the failure is usually attributed to the inexorable consequence of the disease. This type of analysis is not peculiar to doctors, but has graver consequences in medicine than in most fields.

The patient may recover *despite* the treatment. Finally, there are patients who die because of their treatment.

We have at this point established that

- Many doctors have unrealistic estimates of how diagnostic methods and treatment may affect their patients.
- Diagnosis and treatment are often uncoupled and treatment and a happy outcome are often uncoupled.
- Much of medical testing is predictably tangential to the welfare of the patient and some results in harm. In some circumstances, this is unavoidable; in others, it is avoidable.

We are now in a better position to consider the concepts of diagnostic and therapeutic efficiency, which were introduced in Chapter 3.

$$\frac{\text{Diagnostic}}{\text{efficiency}} = \frac{\text{Number of times the test provides an accurate diagnosis}}{\text{Total number of tests}}$$

A more complex expression should be used for *therapeutic* efficiency.

$$\frac{\text{Therapeutic}}{\text{efficiency}} = \frac{\text{Number of effective decisions} - f(\text{mishaps}) + f'(\text{unexpected bonuses})}{\text{Number of tests}}$$

The "number of effective decisions," of course, refers to the number of times the test contributes to better care for the patient. "Mishaps" refers to the number of patients harmed by the given test. The f stands for *function*, meaning that it is difficult to ascribe a specific number to this factor. For example, if a test causes the death of a patient, f should be high. If the mishap is minor, then f should be low.

"Unexpected bonuses" refers to the potential that almost all tests have for producing unexpected results that may benefit the patient. For example, a liver biopsy is performed on a patient who is jaundiced and appears to have infectious hepatitis, which is a viral infection of the liver. There is no specific indication for performing the liver biopsy, as the treatment for infectious hepatitis is nonspecific. Unexpectedly, the liver biopsy reveals the presence of amebiasis, an infection of the liver for which there *is* a specific treatment. The liver biopsy has provided an unexpected but important bonus for one patient.

Again, the f stands for function, meaning that it is difficult to ascribe a specific number to this factor. The existence of unexpected bonuses highlights an important issue: If every conceivable test were performed on every patient, undoubtedly some unsuspected diagnoses would be uncovered that could then be treated with benefit to the patient. This approach is, of course, impractical. Moreover, on balance, more patients unquestionably would be harmed than would benefit.

What you, as a patient, should be interested in is therapeutic efficiency and not diagnostic efficiency. If the results of a test will not benefit you directly, you should be unwilling to undergo the test.

The alarming fact is that, for most tests in medicine, we have no acceptable information on either diagnostic efficiency or therapeutic efficiency. Thus, a whole host of procedures, some of them highly invasive and with the potential to be life-threatening, are performed almost routinely. Many of these can be justified under specific conditions for specific patients. However, their use is substantially more general than can be justified.

We must now ask whether excessive testing per se has the potential to injure patients or whether it is like chicken soup: It either helps or, at worst, does no harm. Actually, an overabundance of tests tends to distract the doctor. He may become so inundated with information that he fails to focus on the problems that are of most concern to the patient. At the least, excessive testing creates unnecessary expense for the patient (or for society); at the most, it causes harm to the patient.

Overtesting

It is easier for doctors to come up with a justification for doing a given test than for not doing it. As the risks of most tests are often not emphasized, errors of commission are more common than errors of omission. The tendency to overtest is so florid that occasionally the physician does not remember whether he ordered a test. The patient charts at a hospital are so crowded with test results that it is easy for a doctor to overlook some.

A consultant, asked to see a patient with a peculiar neurological disorder, was unable to throw light on the neurological disease, but in going over the hospital record he noted that a lung scan had been performed. A lung scan is a test to help diagnose emboli (blood clots) in the lung. There was nothing in the clinical record to suggest such a diagnosis, but the test was positive, indicating that the patient might have emboli in the lung. None of the five doctors who made up the team caring for the patient could come up with a reason for ordering the scan. In fact, none of them recalled ordering the test. They were also unaware that the test was positive.

The consultant speculated that the patient might have cancer of the lung, which is a rare cause of a positive lung scan. If so, the neurological abnormalities might also have been related to cancer of the lung. The consultant then committed a serious error. He discussed the possibility of a diagnosis of lung cancer with the patient and his wife. He then visited the laboratory to inspect the actual lung scan. Here he discovered that there were two patients in the hospital with the same name. The test had been correctly ordered and carried out, but for the other patient. (The other patient did have blood clots in the lung and, for him, the test was appropriate.)

The consultant then returned to his patient and explained his basic error in not checking the original data before causing unnecessary worry and fear. That none of the doctors directly responsible for the care of this patient was surprised that a test, completely tangential to the care of their patient, had been ordered and performed was remarkable. Nor did any of them pay any attention to the results of the test.

The Impact of New Technology

An important question: Has the flood of new technology now available for diagnostic tests improved the outcome of patient management? Superficially it would seem the answer should be yes. A 20-year study, however, concluded that the answer may be no. While the diagnostic tools are getting "better," or at least more sophisticated and costly, the diagnostic results may actually be getting worse. Using a postmortem examination as the gold standard for diagnosis, it was found that in 1960, in about 8 percent of patients who died, doctors had missed problems for which treatment might have resulted in survival; in 1980, this rose to about 10 percent. The study was particularly useful since it addressed the impact of tests on patient welfare and not on diagnosis as an isolated goal.

The problem is not in technological advances per se, but in the system by which new advances are incorporated into medical practice. You will find a discussion of this subject in Chapter 8.

The last quarter-century has seen high technology increasingly introduced into medicine, but the process of evaluating new technological approaches has not changed appreciably. As a result, many tests based on new technology have not been properly evaluated and, in fact, may be useless or harmful.

Guarding Against Overtesting

As a patient, what can you do to avoid excessive testing? Try not to consult doctors for trivial matters. The risks of a needless visit to the doctor are greater than the risks of overlooking an important and treatable disease by staying away.

If your doctor does not volunteer the information, ask what tests are planned and why; try to understand at least the reason why the test is ordered. Do not equate the excellence of a doctor with the number or the complexity or the cost of tests that he orders.

None of these suggestions are absolute safeguards, but the more you understand about the intimate details of your clinical management, the more you can help shape it to meet your needs.

5

The Doctor as God

Healers of all types have often been regarded as possessing mystical powers; the belief that doctors are gods is ancient. To some extent, this has reflected another belief—that illness is a form of divine punishment. Small wonder, then, that divine intervention is required. A modified version of this belief still strongly affects doctor-patient relationships and is often nourished by doctors themselves, not entirely from arrogance or ego, although these may be important factors. The doctor's aura of omniscience fosters feelings of security in the patient. Who wants a doctor who is prone to human error?

This chapter will deal with the risks and benefits of regarding doctors as gods. The following story may be an appropriate introduction: A doctor died and went to heaven, where he found a long line of applicants being screened for admission by St. Peter. Pushing his way to the front of the line, he demanded to be admitted immediately. "I'm sorry," said St. Peter, "but everyone has to wait his turn." Disgruntled, he returned to the end of the line. A figure in a white coat with a stethoscope in his pocket appeared, made his way to the front of the line, and was immediately admitted. Indignant, the doctor complained to St. Peter, "You made me wait and let him in without waiting." "Oh," replied St. Peter, "that's God. He's always playing doctor."

The essence of this story is the perceived arrogance and pretensions of doctors. How arrogant can doctors be? Judge for yourself.

A leading doctor no longer recommends or provides long-term treatment with oxygen for any patient with low blood oxygen levels and chronic lung disease if that patient continues to smoke cigarettes—a surprising position for a doctor to take. It is generally agreed that oxygen treatment improves the quality of life, and perhaps the length of life, in patients with chronic lung disease whether they smoke or not. But he withholds oxygen from these particular patients because he concludes that they will not be helped by oxygen if they continue to smoke.

The doctor's conclusion is based on a study he himself directed. As reported in the medical literature this study showed that recalcitrant smokers continued to have abnormally high numbers of red blood cells despite oxygen treatment, whereas those who saw the light and gave up smoking had closer to normal levels of red blood cells.

His study, of course, failed to address the pertinent question. Do recalcitrant patients who continue to smoke do better on oxygen than recalcitrant patients who are not given oxygen? Do they live longer or better or more productively? One suspects that they do. In addition, there are many recalcitrant smokers who do not have abnormally high numbers of red cells in the blood. Presumably, oxygen treatment will be denied them as well.

From the scientific standpoint, the conclusions do not fit the data. A laboratory test—the measurement of the number of red cells in the blood—is inappropriately used as a substitute for data that would decisively indicate whether or not oxygen treatment is helpful to the patient.

The recommendation to withhold oxygen is particularly ironic. One of the mechanisms by which smoking is said to injure these patients is to increase the amount of carbon monoxide in the blood. Carbon monoxide is one of the products of cigarette smoke inhaled by smokers and interferes with the delivery of oxygen to various tissues of the body. Increases in carbon monoxide in the blood are particularly devastating to those who start out with low oxygen values in the blood. An important form of treatment for carbon monoxide poisoning is breathing high levels of oxygen. Thus, the impact of the recommendation is to deny treatment to those patients who might benefit most from it.

To allow a recalcitrant smoker to die prematurely by depriving him of oxygen would amount to capital punishment. Shades of Gilbert and Sullivan—the punishment would not seem to "fit the crime."

My analysis has been harsh in its judgment. Now let us see if we can determine the reasons for the opinions of the expert. He is a highly respected, well-motivated person. But he has been trained in a profession that encourages arrogance. Individuals in a position to make life-or-death decisions often feel that they have some intrinsic right to do so.

His professional duties require the use of laboratory tests. He is therefore unduly susceptible to asking, "What are the results of a test?" rather than a more important question, "What is the outcome of a given form of therapy for the patient in real life?"

With regard to the particular issue, a personal experience helped shape the views and dictate the godlike decisions of this physician. Some years before, he had been responsible for the care of a patient who was receiving oxygen from a tank. The patient lit a cigarette and was incinerated. (Although oxygen is not flammable, it vigorously supports combustion.) His general upbringing, his training, and his specific experience shaped his opinions. That is to say, he acted as we all do, as a human and not as a god. This, of course, is of scant comfort to patients who might be harmed by his recommendations.

Finally, his opinions were published in an important medical journal and will influence other doctors who may in turn withhold oxygen treatment from patients most in need of it. As we shall see in Chapter 8, the harm that may be done can extend well beyond the immediate sphere of activities of any one doctor.*

Sitting in Judgment

There are various circumstances in which physicians try to behave as gods. An individual doctor may sit in judgment on the social habits of a patient and, in so doing, modify the intensity of care provided. Here is one such instance.

A 57-year-old severe alcoholic is admitted to a hospital in incipient liver coma, a state of depressed mental function caused by severe liver disease. During a discussion to determine what means should be used to treat the patient, one doctor suggests that the treatment not be very intense. This suggestion is put forward, not in the interest of patient comfort or because the patient is dying; rather, it is implied that the patient, being an alcoholic, is really not a very worthwhile member of society. Therefore, why waste the effort and the resources?

What can be said? I think we all expect doctors to do their best for all patients. After all, alcoholism is not a crime. Even if it were, capital punishment seems harsh.

A medical resident refuses to treat a patient with chronic lung disease because the patient will not stop smoking. If the patient continues to smoke, it will undo all of the worthy efforts of the doctor. Why should the doctor bother? Note that the attitude of the resident differs from that of the doctor in the other episode concerning recalcitrant smokers. In this example, the doctor is making a social judgment. In the previous example, the doctor at least used a "scientific" rationalization.

A 20-year-old feeble-minded patient, suffering from chronic kidney failure, was refused treatment with kidney dialysis by a committee set up to judge such matters. At present, the government pays for much of dialysis and, with adequate funds available, many of the ethical problems of select-

*Of course, the author is not a god either and his opinions could be wrong. You will have to decide for yourself.

ing patients seem to have disappeared. Nearly every severely ill patient with kidney disease is eligible. In fact, government support has created a new industry, dialysis for profit. But this incident occurred at a time when the facilities for dialysis were limited and some type of priority system was used to select patients.

The justification for rejecting the patient was that, being feeble-minded, he was not a productive member of society. The young man's minister and his family urged that he be accepted for dialysis. They pointed out that he was deeply religious and, despite the fact that he was feeble-minded, led a happy life. He loved and was loved by his family. The refusal to admit him to the dialysis program amounted to a sentence of death.

The impasse was broken by the intercession of a highly placed doctor who insisted that the young man be accepted for dialysis. The patient was finally treated appropriately because of this doctor's superior firepower.

The New Morality

In recent years, a new version of the old religious doctrine that man's ills are punishment for sin has taken hold in medicine. Disease may now be viewed as a form of punishment for not leading a "good life." Failure to exercise, to eat a proper diet, and to refrain from smoking or drinking are sins punishable by disability or death. Patients who have heart attacks are suffering a form of punishment that could have been avoided by leading a good life—the modern equivalent of doing good deeds.

As a result of this missionary zeal, patients who develop illnesses that could have been avoided by "clean living" feel guilty. Doctors who are true believers tend to look down on the "sinners," exhorting healthy persons to lead a proper life and avoid the fate of those who stray from righteousness. Most of these doctrines do not have a firm scientific basis. There is no question that abstaining from smoking helps to conserve life and that excessive or inappropriate drinking is bad. The value of the rest of the advice is moot. Nevertheless many doctors believe, and preach, that the road to good health is paved with good living habits.

Doctors as Humans

It does not require deep insight to establish that doctors are nongods. Gods do not have high rates of alcoholism, drug addiction, or suicide. Doctors do. Gods are not subject to fatigue nor do they succumb to human foibles. Doctors are and do. The central difference is that gods never make mistakes. Doctors frequently do. And patients must accept an unpleasant fact: Mistakes are an inevitable part of medical care. No doctor has ever practiced error-free medicine. Often mistakes are trivial; at other times, monumental. They may be errors of commission or of omission, errors of judgment, or errors of carelessness. The errors may be avoidable or inevitable, systematic or individual, recognized or unrecognized.

The physician can respond to his perceived mistakes in various ways. The most constructive would be to acknowledge that mistakes are an integral part of medical practice. This would provide a realistic background for dealing with patients. An ongoing critical analysis of the management of individual patients could serve both the doctor and the patient well. A determination to learn from specific errors would make better physicians of us all. A famous clinician once said that he had forgotten many of his triumphs but had never forgotten a single error. He attributed his professional success to learning from his errors. Despite the hyperbole, the lesson is a good one.

The Doctor-as-God Syndrome: Risks Versus Benefits

Now we should analyze the risks and benefits of regarding the doctor as a god. The benefits to the doctor are considerable: It feeds the ego and, in fact, the doctor may begin to believe that he is godlike. It makes patients amenable to his management, so that he does not have to waste time explaining his decisions to them. It binds the patient firmly to the doctor; there is little doctor shopping by patients who deify their doctor.

To the doctor, most of the risks appear to be minor and subtle. In medicine, analysis of errors can be a valuable learning experience, but doctors do not tend toward self-criticism. Godlike status confers on the doctor responsibility for outcome—which he may be unwilling to accept. But on balance, doctors probably feel that the benefits outweigh the risks.

For the patient, the major benefit is a lessening of anxiety. Confidence in the doctor helps create a more favorable atmosphere for recovery. It also shifts the responsibility for management completely to the doctor.

The risks for the patient are considerable. Unquestioning faith in the doctor may give rise to unwarranted expectations and eventual disappointment. And the gulf established between god and mere mortal inhibits the adequate flow of information from doctor to patient. One physician described her mother as an intelligent woman whose intelligence quotient dropped sharply when she consulted a physician. She always left the doctor's office with a series of instructions and medications without understanding what the medications were and why they were given.

The doctor-as-god syndrome is the creation not only of the doctor but also of the patient. In fact, thoughtful doctors have no wish to assume the responsibility of making godlike decisions. Patients frequently leave the doctor no choice. Having projected onto him godlike powers, patients hope to escape responsibility for the outcome of treatment.

Patients are markedly ambivalent toward their doctors. While sick, they commonly attribute godlike qualities to them. When well, they are apt to express a less favorable estimate. Illness for all of us is a time of deep insecurity, and we react to our feelings in various ways. Many seek a figure who can make decisions for them, manage their lives, relieve their doubts, and allay their fears. The doctor as a god often emerges as such a figure.

Occasionally, patients tend to conceal symptoms and signs for fear that these may seem to embody some implicit criticism of the doctor. Their confidence in the godlike doctor sometimes causes patients to deprive themselves of more expert care. On balance, for the patient the risks of regarding doctors as gods considerably outweigh the benefits.

Remember that your doctor is a human and if you treat him like one he is more likely to treat you like one.

6

The Good That Medicine Does

The conquest of poliomyelitis, the near-eradication of tuberculosis, the development of safe and effective surgery in many diseases, the effective treatment of pneumonia, the dramatic advances in the treatment of diabetes and literally hundreds of other diseases—all this is well known. Advances such as these depend upon three elements: (1) an original discovery by a single scientist or a relatively small group of scientists, (2) a health care system capable of quickly translating the discovery into common usage for masses of sick people, and (3) individual doctors who apply the treatment to individual patients.

The Best Game in Town

I hope to convince you that, if you are truly sick, your best course is to consult a medical doctor. Although the conventional health care system has serious flaws, it is "the best game in town."

I will not be able to prove this. This could be done only by setting up alternative health care approaches, applying them to equal numbers of carefully matched cases, and then determining which approach resulted in the best outcome for patients. Such an experiment is impractical. Let us, however, look at two examples that show how well our medical care system can function.

Heart-Lung Transplantation

A 47-year-old woman has a dread disease called primary pulmonary hypertension, meaning that she has high blood pressure in the blood vessels of the lung. As a result, her heart is overworked and has started to fail. As her heart fails, she begins to die. She cannot perform normal physical activity and even talking is difficult. Her tissues are waterlogged, her liver and kidneys no longer function normally, and, as she deteriorates, her life becomes progressively more miserable. She does retain her basic personality; she is an independent, delightful, strong, and somewhat feisty person. She has close and warm family ties and is highly respected in the small community in which she lives.

A team of doctors at a medical center has developed a possible new therapeutic approach to her disease. This approach is heart-lung transplantation—the replacement of her heart and lungs with those of a donor, often an accident victim whose brain is dead but whose heart and lungs are still alive.

The scientific justification for the treatment is provided by a study of a series of monkeys, all of whom were subjected to heart-lung transplantation, the heart and lungs having been obtained from other monkeys. Some of these monkeys have been kept alive for long periods by suppressing their immune processes in order to prevent rejection of new organs. In particular, a new drug, cyclosporin-A, appears to be effective in preventing rejection. This drug has its dangers; it injures the kidneys and the liver and may cause high blood pressure or lymphoma (cancer of the lymph tissue) in a substantial percentage of those receiving it.

The results in the monkey series are not unequivocally favorable. A number of the animals have died because of technical difficulties associated with the heart-lung transplantation. Rejection of the transplanted heart and lungs has occurred in some of the animals; and others have died of miscellaneous causes. But the results are sufficiently promising. A committee of faculty members who attempt to protect the rights of patients being considered for experimental studies is convinced that the procedure should be permitted in humans.

Heart-lung transplantation is offered to our patient. The associated risks and dangers are explained at length and with complete honesty. In fact, the handling of the patient by the surgical team and their assistants is a model of honest human interaction.

The patient accepts the procedure. A donor becomes available. The surgery is performed. The patient survives the surgery. Her postoperative course is difficult; she develops pulmonary edema (extra water in the lung); she has various infections; there is bleeding at the site of surgery and additional surgery is required.

The team of surgeons who look after her believes in doing only what they consider necessary for patient care. They are not addicted to overtesting or overtreatment. She survives and the results are spectacular. She is alive more than two years after the heart-lung transplantation. She has returned to work and is a functioning, vibrant, productive, independent human being. When asked what she most values about the change in her life following the transplantation, she answers, "I can sing with my family."

Literally hundreds of medical advances made this miracle possible: Safe and effective anesthesia, technical expertise to design and perform the surgery, the heart-lung machine that made the surgery practicable, adequate and safe blood replacement, antibiotics to treat infection, drugs to prevent the new heart and lungs from being rejected by the immune system of the host, the use of animals to provide pilot studies, the devoted attention of the team of doctors who cared for the patient—even the ability of medicine to find a donor and to locate this single heroic patient were made possible by our health care system.

Near-Drowning

A 3-year-old girl is found face down in a swimming pool by her mother. The child is not breathing and her heart may have stopped. Her mother uses cardiopulmonary resuscitation (CPR); the child begins to breathe and her heart starts to beat. Help is summoned and the patient is transported to a hospital.

Her course in the hospital is stormy and prolonged. She is comatose for a number of days, and it is feared that she has suffered permanent brain damage from lack of oxygen during the episode of near-drowning. She also has a variety of lung infections. In addition, as is common in these patients, there is evidence of severe lung injury. The patient requires a breathing machine, or ventilator, to maintain adequate lung function and continuous oxygen administration. There are numerous complications, and a team of doctors provides constant care in an attempt to keep her alive. Her father and her mother also devote full time to her. Despite this, it is the impression of her doctors that she is going downhill and will probably die.

An outside consultant is asked to see the child to determine whether anything more can be done to halt her deterioration. In particular, he is asked whether she should be treated with an artificial lung. Such an experimental machine is available less than 50 miles away.

The consultant suggests three things. One is not to abandon hope—as to the general outcome, as to whether the brain is permanently damaged, or as to whether the lung injury will be fatal. In his opinion, any judgments on these problems are premature. He also advises strongly against the use of the experimental artificial lung. Data available to him suggest that this approach is not likely to be helpful and, in fact, may be harmful. Since only a limited data base is available, he considers that the risks are enormous and the benefits are dubious. His best opinion is to not use this form of therapy.

He suggests a new and untested form of therapy, the administration of two enzymes that can be instilled in the patient's lungs and that, theoretically, might be helpful in over-coming the progressive lung deterioration. But he emphasizes that there is no acceptable scientific basis for their use. However, his feeling is that, unlike the lung machine, these agents, even if they prove useless, will probably not harm her. He considers the risks to be minimal and, even if the benefits are also minimal, the risk-benefit ratio is acceptable. In addition, he knows that it is important for the family and the medical staff to feel that no potentially helpful therapy is being over-looked.

His advice is accepted and the enzymes are obtained and used. The patient begins to improve. The improvement is not rapid or dramatic. In the opinion of some physicians, the enzyme therapy played an important role. Others feel that the improvement was not related to the use of the new drugs. The consultant concurs in the latter opinion.

Over a period of months, the patient gradually recovers. Discharged from the hospital, she undergoes an intensive period of rehabilitation at home. Five years later, as of this writing, she is a lovely, talented, and, understandably, moderately spoiled young lady.

Cardiopulmonary Resuscitation(CPR)

The use of cardiopulmonary resuscitation (CPR) was the initial and essential first step. CPR, developed by doctors and widely used by para-medical personnel and the lay public, has saved an enormous number of lives. The actual mechanism by which CPR causes the heart to pump blood is not known. This does not detract from its utility. There are many therapeutic approaches in medicine in which the mechanism of action is not known. This does not matter to patients; what matters is whether or not they work.

Should we apply a risk-benefit analysis to CPR? For most patients, the answer is obviously no. Failure to maintain breathing and heart action means death in a short period of time. Such well-documented risks of CPR as rib fracture or rupture of an internal organ are trivial in comparison with the possible saving of a life.

There are patients in whom CPR is inappropriate. Patients with brain death, or with far advanced cancer or certain neurological diseases, are commonly considered "no code." This means that if the heart stops or the patient stops breathing in the hospital, no effort is made to resuscitate them. In such patients, it has already been determined that the benefits of continued life are negligible. As you may imagine, to classify a patient "no code" is not an easy decision.

Risk-benefit analysis is also more difficult in patients with prolonged cessation of heartbeat or breathing. There may already be irreversible changes in brain function even if the patient does not die quickly. If such patients are resuscitated, they may survive indefinitely but without brain function. Minimizing this risk is very difficult. It is estimated that the average time following arrest of the *heart* before death occurs is about four minutes; the average time following arrest of *breathing* before death occurs might be eight minutes. But these estimates are not necessarily applicable, because it is seldom possible to fix the time of the onset of cardiac arrest or the cessation of breathing. And not every case conforms to the estimates. Survival with preservation of brain function has been described following even 15 minutes of apparent cardiac arrest. Successful resuscitation and salvage have been described at very low temperatures—for example, in drowning children, even after several hours of submersion in icy water. In fact, it was knowledge of this that led to the hope that irreversible changes in brain function had not occurred in our patient.

The instinctive reaction of the mother of our patient was consistent with present knowledge. Conventional practice is to use CPR unless, and until, it is clear that there are powerful reasons for not doing so. A patient whose heart is not beating, or who is not breathing, should not be the subject of a careful risk-benefit analysis. It is a time to act. CPR was a decisive factor in saving this child's life.

Assessing Modern Medicine

Modern medicine contributed in numerous ways to her survival. Her brain was protected from further deterioration by the use of various drugs. Medical technology provided a ventilator that furnished appropriate amounts of oxygen and permitted adequate excretion of carbon dioxide. Antibiotics were available to treat infection. A devoted medical team treated her vigilantly and a system of medical consultation provided some helpful input. In contrast to the first patient, her life was probably saved by *not* subjecting her to an unproven form of treatment, the artificial lung. Undoubtedly, some measures undertaken were useless and others may have harmed her. But, on the whole, her care was thoughtful and excellent.

If medical care were as excellent on the average as it demonstrably was in these two patients, this book would not have been written. If medical care were as poor on the average as it was in patients described in earlier chapters, this book would be many times its present length. Most medical care falls between these extremes. We can assess the medical system by considering three questions:

- What features of the conventional medical care system account for its strengths?
- What are the alternatives to conventional medical care?
- Can we systematically correct what is bad in patient management? (This question is considered at length in the last chapter and the appendix.)

Strengths of Conventional Medical Care

Let us first consider the strengths of the conventional medical care system. The care that your doctor provides is scientifically based. This cannot be taken to mean that your doctor is a scientist or that medical care is a science, but it does have important positive implications. Your physician's approach to treatment is not based on fixed, invariant, or nondemonstrable assumptions. Doctors require some evidence to justify most important actions.

The doctor's approaches to disease, being scientifically based, change with time as new evidence evolves. This is important because, as you will see, at any one time much of accepted medical knowledge is incorrect. Medicine benefits from new and revolutionary advances in science, and its capacity to change has dividends for patients.

Three scientific revolutions now occurring should lead to substantial advances in patient care. One is the ability to modify genetic processes by manipulating DNA, the chemical blueprints that specify the body's structure and function. So-called genetic engineering is but the tip of this iceberg. Continuing advances in this area can be expected to greatly enlarge our understanding of disease and its treatment.

The transplantation of specific organs constitutes a second revolution. The lives of thousands of patients with kidney disease have already been altered for the better. Lens transplantation has improved the vision of thousands. Heart transplantation, heart-lung transplantation, bone marrow transplantation, and pancreatic transplantation are in their infancy; all will bring even greater benefits. We are probably still in the first stages of learning how to use this tool to improve patient welfare.

The use of computers in medicine has created a third revolution. The capacity for storage and retrieval of information is now enormous, and even this simple application cannot help but improve patient care. Soon the world's knowledge in specific areas of disease will be available to every doctor. As and if artificial intelligence becomes a reality, or even as we improve the information we feed to computers, medicine will take a giant step forward.

As advances like these occur, each is fed into the system of conventional practice and quickly applied. Of course, the price our patients pay is that inadequate and harmful approaches are also fed in quickly, but we can't have it both ways.

Our conventional health care system supports a vast organized communication network. There are innumerable medical journals, medical textbooks, and medical meetings that reach many physicians. Through this network, the experience of small groups of doctors becomes available to doctors generally.

The health care system is structured to provide stability and continuity to health care. The training of physicians follows an organized format, and certain minimal requirements are enforced. Postgraduate training, which is the rule for most doctors, guarantees a graded increase in responsibility before the doctor practices on his own. An extensive hospital system provides not only the facilities for handling patients, but a place for learning and peer review.

Immense support facilities exist for the conventional system. Among them are: A drug industry to seek and develop therapeutic agents (the primary motive is profit but, in general, the industry operates within strict limits); an industrial base for the development of medical technology (it also operates to make money but, in general, it also operates within strict controls); nurses and paramedical personnel, who contribute immeasurably to health care. Every time you consult an individual physician, you also gain entry into the entire system.

The medical care system accepts responsibility for correcting those of its errors that are identified. Some of the problems described in this book are recognized and under close scrutiny. Physicians themselves often take the initiative in attempting to correct errors.

What about the doctor? Physicians are generally concerned and well-motivated people. They have gone through a long period of training in a profession whose tradition emphasizes service to others. The profession does contain (we hope less than) its share of incompetents, psychopaths, misfits, quacks, and simply inadequate individuals. It also has (we hope more than) its share of well-trained, effective, and highly productive people.

There is little question that, on the average, doctors attempt to provide the best care they can for their patients. Even after completing their formal education, the great majority continue to train and to attend postgraduate medical courses. (Perhaps there is a preference for meetings in Florida in the winter and Greece in the summer; why not?) They buy large numbers of medical journals and texts and usually read them. Doctors continue their efforts to improve their technical proficiency, which is usually good and often spectacular.

Alternatives to Conventional Medicine

What are the alternatives to conventional medical care? A variety of approaches are available: Faith healing, religious healing, holistic medicine, acupuncture, chiropractic, and nutrition among them. Some of these are offered by medical doctors; most are not. While I am no expert on these various systems, several things seem clear. Their scientific bases are obscure or nonexistent, and their assumptions are untestable. They do not appear to operate by strict rules of evidence, nor is there an independently verifiable track record. Their infrastructure is rudimentary. There are often no minimal requirements of training or experience for their practitioners. They usually lack any long tradition of care and frequently have little stability. Often when practitioners of these systems become ill, they consult medical doctors.

My opinion is that if you are truly sick you had better go to a medical doctor. Your chances of being helped are substantially greater inside than outside the conventional health care system. Doctors are in general agreement that the vast majority of patients who consult them are not really ill. If that is true of you, your choice of health system will probably make little difference. Assume, however, that you are truly sick. If you consult a conventional practitioner, the odds are that you will be treated by a system whose advantages are proven. If you choose to go outside of the system, you will lose most of these advantages.

Your best bet is to see a doctor. This does not guarantee that you will get the best possible care, but a careful risk-benefit analysis favors the choice of conventional medicine. No vast collection of magical herbs exists out there, unknown to your doctor, to cure your problem. Many patients who find their way into these alternate systems are failures of the conventional system; that is, they have problems that cannot be successfully treated by conventional medicine and are not treatable by any other means.

If you are not very sick, but need emotional support, you will surely find among doctors at least as many compassionate, sensitive, helpful humans as you will find in the alternative forms of health care.

May you always be so well that you never require the services of a doctor. If you do need one, may you be so fortunate that he does you more good than harm.

7

The Harm That Medicine Does— Iatrogenic Episodes

Iatrogenic (Greek, *iatros* = doctor, *genic* = arising from or developing from) literally means disease or illness caused by doctors. This definition, however, is too broad. Almost everything a doctor does has potential risks as well as potential benefits. Should we consider every mishap related to treatment as an iatrogenic episode? No. There are many circumstances in which the doctor deliberately places the patient at risk because the potential benefits outweigh the risks.

A 26-year-old woman develops leukemia, a cancer of the bone marrow; the treatment for this disease is a drug that may cause depression of white blood cells and lower resistance to infection. Her doctor warns her of this possibility. Together they decide that the risk of infection is preferable to the risk of untreated leukemia. With treatment, her white-blood-cell count does indeed drop to a dangerous level and she develops a life-threatening bacterial infection.

A 40-year-old man has cancer of the blood vessels; the treatment for his disease is a drug known to produce serious and occasionally fatal heart disease when used in therapeutic doses. The patient and his doctor both understand and agree to accept the risk. The patient receives the proper dose of the medicine and develops fatal heart disease.

Neither of these can be considered an iatrogenic episode. But what if a patient is accidentally given an overdose of a

74

drug—a dose that *invariably* injures the heart? This would constitute an iatrogenic episode.

Part of the doctor's job is to risk harming patients in order to help them. When he does this consciously and deliberately, with knowledge of the risks but in the belief that the benefits outweigh the risks, even if the patient is harmed, he has not created a mishap.

In an iatrogenic episode a patient is harmed as a result of an error in diagnosis or treatment, or as a result of a mishap during medical care. The harm is independent of the natural progression of the patient's illness and treatment and represents part of the risk that the patient *must* assume as an inevitable component of management. As we will see from the following examples, iatrogenic episodes arise from nonsystematic errors. Such episodes are alarmingly frequent in hospitals.

The Cascade Effect

A young man entered a hospital to be operated on for an ingrown toenail, a trivial but annoying problem. The operation is also relatively trivial. Because the patient was apprehensive, it was decided to put him to sleep for the procedure. While the anesthesia was being administered, the patient's heart stopped. The surgeon opened the chest and succeeded in restarting the heart, but because haste was imperative, failed to take adequate sterile precautions. After resuscitation, while being wheeled to a hospital room, the patient suffered a fractured leg in an elevator accident. He was returned to surgery, where the fractured leg was placed in a cast.

During the course of the next two days, he developed bacterial pericarditis, an infection of the membranes covering the heart, undoubtedly the result of inadequate sterilization at the time his chest was opened to restart his heart. An operation on the heart was now necessary to drain the infection. This was followed by treatment with antibiotics, during which the patient developed a pulmonary embolism or blood clot in the lung, a common complication both of major fractures of the leg and of prolonged bed rest. This in turn required treatment with an anticlotting drug, and massive bleeding from an ulcer in the stomach followed. The ulcer was probably the result of stress related to the numerous complications and treatments he had undergone, and the anticlotting drug increased the intensity of the bleeding.

After some months, the patient was discharged from the hospital, his ingrown toenail still untreated. He left the hospital alive, a tribute to his youth and his indomitable spirit.

This lamentable tale, with its air of gallows humor, is hardly typical. It has great value, however, as an illustration of the process by which "for want of a nail, a shoe was lost; for want of a shoe, the horse was lost; and for want of a horse, the rider was lost." The original error in the treatment of this patient was to use general anesthesia for a trivial surgical procedure. Cardiac arrest or death is rare in these circumstances, but it does occur. An occasional patient dies, for example, during the simple extraction of a tooth. Serious iatrogenic episodes tend to cascade—one complication follows another. As disease becomes more severe, the range and intensity of treatment increases, leading to a greater possibility of iatrogenic episodes.

A 78-year-old woman suffered massive bleeding from the gastrointestinal tract. During treatment, she developed adult respiratory distress syndrome (ARDS), a form of lung disease that commonly occurs in many forms of severe illness. Probably half of the affected patients die because the lungs are unable to absorb adequate amounts of oxygen from inspired air.

The usual treatment is to place the patient on a ventilator and provide air enriched with oxygen. In this patient, even when pure oxygen was administered, the oxygen in the blood stayed at dangerously low levels. The patient's physician knew that in ARDS the inability to oxygenate the lungs with a high concentration of oxygen usually indicates a hopeless prognosis.

He so informed the patient's family and, being a sensitive and excellent practitioner, suggested that all treatment except that required for her comfort be withdrawn. After much soul-searching, the family agreed. The patient was taken off the ventilator and supplemental oxygen and permitted to breathe room air, whereupon the oxygen level in her blood improved significantly. Inspection of the ventilator revealed that one of the valves in the apparatus functioned poorly, so that the patient had been breathing a gas mixture actually lower in oxygen than ordinary room air. How much the exposure to oxygen-poor air contributed to her subsequent death is difficult to judge.

Another 78-year-old woman, previously hale and vigorous, and much loved by her family, developed a respiratory infection. The infection may have been bronchitis, a relatively minor infection of the bronchial tubes, or it may have been pneumonia, a more serious infection of the lung tissue. Neither necessarily requires hospitalization. She was nevertheless admitted to a hospital and during routine testing of her blood was found to have a low potassium level. Although he observed no obvious manifestations of potassium deficiency, her physician prescribed potassium to be administered by vein.

Even in patients with low potassium levels, replacing potassium too rapidly can cause death—potassium intoxication can stop the heart. A potassium solution was administered to this patient, but with inadequate monitoring. Her heart stopped, and postmortem examination of the blood revealed that she had almost certainly died of potassium intoxication. Had she not been admitted to a hospital, she would probably have survived. Had the level of potassium in the blood not been measured, she almost certainly would not have died.

Atropine, a drug used to treat a slow heart rate, was prescribed for a patient suffering from this abnormality. The usual dose is 0.2 milligrams; the drug is packaged in small vials, each containing this dose. A nurse misread the doctor's order, and administered the contents of 20 vials to the patient. What went through her mind as she opened 20 separate vials is difficult to guess. The patient, not surprisingly, developed atropine poisoning; he survived, but only after a stormy course.

A patient with severe gastrointestinal bleeding was to be treated with an antacid delivered through a tube placed directly in the stomach. Antacids are thick, viscous liquids, and should be delivered only directly into the gastrointestinal tract. Another tube for administering intravenous fluids was attached to a needle and inserted into a vein. Somehow the bottles leading to the tubes were interchanged. The antacid was dripped into the veins of the patient, who died of antacid emboli (antacid particles clogging his veins).

A patient with blood type O was mistakenly administered three units of blood type A. He suffered a massive transfusion reaction and died.

Almost every physician can furnish his own chamber of horrors. Their collective frequency represents the degree of potential risk incurred in being treated by doctors. If episodes of this type are common, then the risk is high; if episodes are exceedingly rare, then the risk is small.

Iatrogenic Risk-Benefit Analysis of Hospitalization

A large-scale study examined the hospital records of 808 consecutive admissions to a university hospital medical ward. The results were staggering. Roughly one-third of the patients admitted had developed either a major or minor complication associated with treatment. In 8 percent of the patients these were major complications, defined as mishaps that were potentially life-threatening. In 2 percent of the patients, the iatrogenic episode contributed directly to the patient's death.

Admittedly, the design of this study was poor. It was retrospective—that is, the hospital records were surveyed after the patients were discharged or died—and retrospective studies are notoriously inaccurate. The records were painstakingly scrutinized and perhaps even the most trivial iatrogenic episodes were detected. Furthermore, these 808 patients may not have been truly representative of the entire population of hospitalized patients. But, even allowing for its imperfections, the study shows that the incidence of iatrogenic episodes is discouragingly high. The cases cited in this chapter, while not necessarily typical of hospital care, are probably not unusual.

"Desperate diseases require desperate measures." In the attempt to save patients who might otherwise die, doctors are required to use heroic measures and multiple interventions. The same study revealed that the frequency of iatrogenic episodes was even greater in the critically ill. (The incidence of life-threatening mishaps was about 25 percent.) The more that is done to patients and the more aggressive the treatment, the greater the risks and the possibility of mishaps. This is not, however, the complete explanation. Desperate measures are commonly used when lesser measures would be more appropriate. Doctors may fail to recognize that nondesperate diseases require nondesperate measures.

It would be reassuring to know that, on balance, more critically ill patients are helped than harmed. This may be so, but it has by no means been established. The old bromide that we doctors bury our mistakes contains some truth. In the absence of any general systematic attempt to collect data on iatrogenic episodes, doctors underestimate the incidence of iatrogenic episodes.

In making a risk-benefit analysis, we can take it as a given that the risks of hospitalization are high in terms of iatrogenic episodes. How shall we estimate the benefits? Put another way, how sick should one be to enter a hospital? We can begin by asking what percentage of hospitalizations are unnecessary. If the percentage is high, then the risk-benefit ratio of hospitalization is unfavorable for those patients who are hospitalized unnecessarily. If, on the other hand, most hospital admissions are necessary, then the risk-benefit ratio is more favorable.

There is something to be learned from other countries. In

several health care systems outside the United States, the rate of hospitalization per unit of population is approximately half that of the United States. Despite this, the death rate per unit of population in these countries compares favorably with ours. This suggests—although it does not prove—that a substantial percentage of hospital admissions in the United States may be unnecessary and that the risk-benefit ratio of hospitalization for many patients is therefore unacceptably high.

What do doctors do to minimize iatrogenic episodes? Actually, very little. American hospitals traditionally conduct morbidity and mortality conferences at which the medical staff discusses what went wrong with selected patients. These are usually desultory analyses; they cover only a few patients and have little impact. The only, or best, records of the mishaps that occur are commonly the nurses' notes on hospital charts.

Some hospitals conduct reviews of the quality of patient care. Interestingly enough, reviews focus on procedures that were *not* performed in the care of specific diseases. They almost never focus on what *was* done that was improper: "Doctor Jones did *not* order lung function studies in a patient with lung disease" rather than "Doctor Jones gave a tranquilizer to a patient with lung disease, which precipitated respiratory failure and killed the patient." The effect of these reviews is to create more overtesting and overtreatment, rather than less.

Because the attempt to detect and eliminate iatrogenic episodes in out-patient practice is even less developed than in hospitals, less is known about their prevalence outside hospitals. As a result, doctors practice in an atmosphere of unrealistic self-confidence. We doctors are all aware that serious errors arise in patient care, but it is usually someone else's patient who is harmed.

Some Measures to Decrease Iatrogenics

What could the medical system do to decrease the incidence of iatrogenic episodes?

Medical schools can begin by teaching students to recognize iatrogenic episodes, to deal with them, and to learn from them. Students would come to know how much vigilance is required to decrease their number, how to avoid unnecessary hospitalizations, and how to avoid unnecessary or overly aggressive diagnostic and therapeutic procedures.

The modern medical school does alert students to the dangers of various drugs and procedures. But this aspect of their training tends to be buried in a mass of other details, so that medical students leave school overly impressed with the beneficial effects of the skills they have acquired and too little aware of their capacity to do harm. A more realistic balance would be achieved in a less self-congratulatory atmosphere.

Hospitals should take major responsibility for decreasing iatrogenic episodes

- By making an organized effort to discourage unnecessary admissions—at present they are making organized attempts to encourage admissions
- By instituting a surveillance and reporting system to quantitate and analyze iatrogenic episodes
- By encouraging self-surveillance and self-analysis by the individual doctor

As a patient, what can you do to protect yourself from iatrogenic episodes? You have already learned that you should avoid unnecessary testing. As the most serious iatrogenic episodes occur in hospitals, you should try to keep out of the hospital. You should agree to hospitalization only when you are seriously ill, or when you require the facilities of a hospital for treatment. If you go to the hospital, insist on spending only as much time there as is absolutely essential for dealing with your specific problem. Remember, too, that the more you know about the details of your management, the better you can protect yourself.

To eliminate iatrogenic episodes entirely is impossible. Given the whims of fate, the complexities of disease, and the nature of human frailties, some mishaps will occur to some patients. The goal of medicine should be to decrease these to an irreducible minimum.

8

The Harm That Medicine Does — Iatroepidemics

Iatroepidemic is a term I have coined to denote an epidemic, or plague, caused by doctors. Like *iatrogenic* it derives from the Greek (*iatros* =doctor, *epi* =on, *demos* =people). Iatroepidemics develop because of systematic errors incorporated into medical practice. The application of these errors to masses of patients results in harm or death to large numbers. Unlike iatrogenic episodes, which are random and accidental, iatroepidemics are systematic and their causes are predictable—and therefore potentially preventable.

In recognizing and admitting past errors, medicine could hope to establish a process for identifying and correcting current errors. The Nobel Laureate and physicist Max Planck described the process by which science advances: "A new scientific truth does not triumph by convincing its opponents and making them see the light, but rather because its opponents eventually die and a new generation grows up that is familiar with it." Medicine too often follows the same pattern and at a terrible cost. Too many patients have died before the proponents of the old "truths." Planck's description applies perfectly to the story of Semmelweis and childbed fever.

Puerperal (Childbed) Fever

Puerperal fever, more commonly known as childbed fever, was a major cause of death in the nineteenth century; it followed childbirth, often with a rapid and progressive course and death. We now know that the disease was infectious and caused by bacteria, but the germ theory of disease—the concept that germs caused infection and that the infection could be spread from one person to another—had not yet been formulated.

A young Hungarian-born obstetrician, Ignaz Philipp Semmelweis, worked on an obstetrical ward in a famous Viennese hospital, Allgemeines Krankenhaus. His ward was organized so that medical students and faculty came directly from performing autopsies to the ward, where they examined one patient after another, performing vaginal examinations without washing their hands. A second ward was devoted to the training of midwives. The midwives did wash their hands between patients, probably for reasons of personal cleanliness rather than to protect their charges.

Noting that women clamored to be admitted to the midwives' ward rather than the doctors' ward, Semmelweis made a careful study of the autopsy records of patients who had died of puerperal fever. These confirmed the prejudice of the patients—the death rate was astronomical in the doctors' ward, strikingly higher than in the midwives' ward.

The crucial observation came when a colleague died after cutting himself during an autopsy on a patient who had died of puerperal fever. In performing an autopsy on his unfortunate colleague, Semmelweis noted findings indistinguishable from those found in women who died of puerperal fever. He thereupon made the daring guess that his colleague, though male, had actually died of childbed fever. This led him to a series of deductions:

- Puerperal fever was somehow carried to the patients who developed the disease, perhaps from another patient.
- The carrier of the disease was often the doctor himself.

- Transmission of the disease could be limited by simple hygienic practices, such as washing one's hands before performing a vaginal examination.

Semmelweis had no idea that germs caused the disease, no tests to detect the disease in its earliest phase, and no firm evidence that his theories were correct; he simply put together a series of brilliant intuitions. Thereafter he insisted that everyone handling deliveries on his ward wash their hands in a chemical solution before examining any patient. The death rate on his ward dropped dramatically.

Semmelweis published his views in the medical literature and met with fierce opposition from orthodox obstetricians, especially from the leaders among them. Driven from Vienna, he returned to Budapest, where he continued to fight orthodoxy. His opponents were relentless; he was attacked not only medically and scientifically, but personally as well. Some individual doctors supported him openly or in spirit, but the nature of medicine is such that modes of practice are set by influential experts. When they are wrong, they carry the bulk of doctors along with them. So it was in this case.

History records that his sensitive nature could not withstand the assault. He brooded over numerous wrongs, went insane, and died. But his views eventually triumphed. With the institution of hygienic practices, puerperal fever virtually disappeared, and millions of pregnant women owe a debt of gratitude to this pioneer.

What can we say of this story, 140 years later, in the light of our present knowledge? First, that the episode was truly an iatroepidemic; doctors themselves literally spread death. That they themselves might be the instruments by which patients were harmed was inconceivable. His opponents were undoubtedly convinced that they were practicing excellent obstetrics. It would have been especially galling to suffer by comparison to "mere" midwives. The very idea that they, doctors, were responsible for spreading disease and death was undoubtedly too repugnant a notion for them to consider. Their abuse of Semmelweis can be seen as an overreaction to this threat to their self-esteem.

If we were to look for some justification for their actions, we would have to know how many crackpot schemes were rejected in the nineteenth century because the leaders of medicine were not quick to accept new ideas. Medical conservatism may serve to protect patients as well as to harm them. This justification, however, does not withstand critical analysis. None of the experts approached the problem by saying, "We will stay with the old ways until there is firm proof." Nor would they have thought of setting up an experiment in which half of the women were delivered by "clean" doctors and the other half by "dirty" doctors. Semmelweis's opinions were rejected out of hand, even though what he proposed was, in retrospect, so trivial—washing one's hands in a solution of calcium chloride. In terms of risk-benefit analysis, there was almost no risk in trying Semmelweis's approach.

Why do we honor Semmelweis? Because he was right. His views ultimately saved millions of lives. Although the scientific basis of his approach, the germ theory of disease, was not established until 25 years later, he dared to trust his analysis. We also admire his courage and tenacity; the fact that he may have died because of his opinions seems only to increase our admiration.

What can be learned from this dramatic story? Experts resist change. There was no immediate mass conversion of obstetricians to hygienic practice, and it is probable that pregnant women continued to die needlessly long after Semmelweis's views became widely accepted. Medicine, like other areas of human behavior, has long cultural lags. As we look back 140 years later, can we be certain that the equivalent of Semmelweis's views would fare better today? Are new ideas more acceptable today, when a correct theory can be more rapidly translated into general use?

Radical Mastectomy

From 1907 until 1955, radical mastectomy was virtually mandatory treatment for cancer of the breast. In this operation not only the breast but much of the surrounding tissue is removed. The surgeon who introduced the operation justified it on two grounds: First, it seemed reasonable to assume that the more tissue was removed, the greater the likelihood that all of the cancerous tissue would be excised. Second, it seemed reasonable to assume that the cancer would always spread directly from its original or local site to the surrounding tissue —a view now known to be naive and incorrect. The adoption of radical mastectomy was not based on careful studies demonstrating that patients fared better after radical mastectomy than after less radical forms of surgery. (We should not be too critical, however. The requirement for this kind of evidence was simply not part of established medicine in 1907.)

Radical mastectomy became the accepted form of treatment for cancer of the breast, and by 1955 huge numbers of women had undergone this physically and psychologically mutilating operation. Reluctant patients were informed that without a radical mastectomy, they would almost certainly die of cancer. Not many resisted when offered a choice between disfigurement and death.

In 1955, a surgeon suggested that simple circumscribed excision of the cancer (lumpectomy) followed by x-ray treatment was as effective as radical mastectomy. The basis for his claim was more valid than that for the surgical introduction of radical mastectomy. He had tested his idea in a clinical trial on a small series of patients and found that they did as well as those treated with radical mastectomy. But his views were not accepted. (He may not have been the first to provide data questioning the need for radical mastectomy. Similar results obtained by other surgeons were also either ignored or discounted.) Nevertheless, he has continued to the present time to treat patients by the less drastic procedures he advocates. And he has been vindicated.

During the past decade substantial data have accumulated to show that, in the case of localized breast cancer, lumpectomy followed by x-ray produces survival rates not significantly different from those of radical mastectomy. Lumpectomy plus radiation is now medically respectable. Thousands of women are being spared a physically and emotionally damaging procedure, because radical mastectomy is no longer considered the only acceptable form of treatment.

The issue is not completely resolved. Some experts claim that after 15 to 20 years, patients treated with radical mastectomy show a slightly higher survival rate than those treated with lumpectomy and radiation. This claim is usually made by surgeons. It is more or less a general rule of iatroepidemics that the specialist whose practice is being challenged—the one whose "ox is gored"—leads the defense of the old practice. It seems clear, however, that the failure to consider alternate forms of therapy in 1955 deprived countless women of a choice that is now acceptable. Had radical mastectomy been subjected to a clinical trial in 1955, many would doubtless have been spared this disfiguring and traumatic treatment.*

Spurious Pulmonary Embolism

The following account is detailed and complicated. You may want to skip it or skim it and come back to it later. It is not essential to your grasp of the chapter, but it is instructive.

Pulmonary embolism (clots in the blood vessels of the lung) is a common disease that can lead to death by causing abnormalities of heart and/or lung function. It is usually seen in patients who are at high risk because of prolonged bed rest, prolonged automobile trips, pregnancy, fractured legs, sur-

---

*In fact, some experts now claim that up to 80 percent of women with breast cancer should be treated with radiation alone.

gery, heart failure, perhaps the use of birth control pills, increases in blood count, and chronic illness. Previously normal subjects without obvious risk factors may also develop the disease.

Pulmonary embolism resembles a number of other common diseases affecting the lungs. The clinical findings may be similar to those in patients with heart attacks, lung infection, collapsed lung, and pleural infection (the pleura are the membranes covering the lung). As the combined total number of patients with these diseases is substantially greater than the number of those with pulmonary embolism, the possibilities for overdiagnosis are great.

For the patient, the stakes in an accurate diagnosis are very high. A false-negative patient is deprived of proper treatment. Patients with pulmonary embolism should be treated with anticoagulants, agents which prevent clotting of the blood. Otherwise, these patients may die or be disabled.

A false-positive diagnosis is also dangerous: Anticoagulants can cause disability or fatal bleeding. Grave life-style consequences follow a diagnosis of pulmonary embolism: The patient may be needlessly impoverished by giving up a job because of a disease he does not have; he may no longer be insurable. Women who want children may be dissuaded from having them because of the fear of recurrence, while women who do not want children may be taken off birth control pills, as the use of the pills may be related to pulmonary embolism. The patient may be emotionally crippled because of worry about the disease. The term *thromboneurosis* has been coined to describe this outcome.

A small percentage of patients who actually have pulmonary embolism ultimately develop a chronic disease, pulmonary hypertension (high blood pressure in the blood vessels of the lung). This is a disabling and frequently fatal disease for which there is no effective treatment—not a worry you would want hanging over you for the rest of your life.

In 1964, a laboratory test for the diagnosis of pulmonary

embolism was introduced. The test is called a perfusion lung scan and uses advanced technology and radioisotopes. The test was developed by experts in nuclear medicine and is performed by specialists in this area. Its accuracy or usefulness was never adequately established; validation consisted of some inadequate animal studies and desultory retrospective studies in patients.

Although a highly accurate existing test, called pulmonary angiography, could have been used to evaluate the validity of the perfusion scan test, this was not done. Probably because it is invasive, inconvenient, and may result in morbidity and even mortality, pulmonary angiography never caught on. But it is the "gold standard" of diagnosis in this disease.

Perfusion lung scans were widely used without adequate validation on hundreds of thousands of patients in this country alone. A major attraction of the test is that it is minimally invasive, requiring only an intravenous injection. Only two deaths have been reported from its use in huge numbers of patients. The test is relatively simple, and the necessary equipment is available at many hospitals.

Noninvasiveness, ease, and safety are often cited as important advantages of tests, but unless a test is accurate, these factors are irrelevant. The perfusion lung scan was widely acclaimed in the medical literature; some doctors built their reputations on it. All of this occurred without acceptable verification and without proof that the test was of any real value. Some doctors were skeptical, but their opinions carried little weight.

In 1971, the nuclear medicine experts introduced a new test called a ventilation scan of the lung to supplement the perfusion lung scan. The alleged value of the ventilation scan was that it increased the specificity of the perfusion lung scan. It would supposedly enable the doctor to discriminate between a true positive, in which the patient actually has a pulmonary embolism, and a false positive, in which the patient does not have a pulmonary embolism. Widely accepted, it was used, like the perfusion lung scan, with inadequate validation. Acceptance of both these tests by physicians was based on faith —a reliance on the experts and on the mystique of advanced technology.

Late in 1977, a dark cloud appeared on the horizon. The accuracy and validity of the diagnostic management of pulmonary embolism were challenged by a lung expert.* He raised several issues. He emphasized the inadequacies of clinical diagnosis. He affirmed the value of a negative perfusion scan in ruling out a diagnosis of pulmonary embolism (adequate sensitivity). However, he criticized the value of a positive perfusion scan, contending that many patients without pulmonary embolism showed positive results (unacceptably low specificity). He contended that a ventilation scan was seldom or never of value in making a positive diagnosis of pulmonary embolism. He concluded that this resulted in major overdiagnosis and overtreatment of the disease.

A national group of nuclear medicine experts, appalled at his questioning of the value of their diagnostic methods, decided on a strategy: They would analyze the records of their home institutions to establish the value of scanning for the diagnosis of pulmonary embolism, and these data would be summarized in a common publication to be signed jointly by all the experts. The effect would be decisive, clearly refuting the maverick expert and establishing beyond question the value of scanning.

You may have guessed what happened. When they went to analyze their records, they found that the cupboard was bare.

*This expert had an interesting history in relation to the diagnosis of pulmonary embolism. Some 20 years earlier he had introduced his own diagnostic test, and it had proved useless. He had made two erroneous assumptions: One, that the clinical diagnosis of pulmonary embolism was reliable; the other, that the findings of the animal studies he used to validate his test were applicable to human patients. Neither assumption was correct. He publicly disavowed his own test. Despite this, some physicians continue to rely on this useless test even today.

There were no data clearly proving the value of the tests. At this point, the nuclear medicine authorities had three choices: They could admit they had no data to support their current practice. This would not necessarily mean that they had been wrong; it would mean that, at worst, they had been careless. This alternative had little appeal. They could organize a proper study to fill the major gap in data that they now knew existed. This they did not do. Finally, they could attack the philistine, using whatever ammunition was available for the purpose. This was the course they selected.

This was a critical time. Before they recognized that they could not validate their practice, the response of the experts was perhaps understandable. Their actions, once they realized that adequate data were not available, were more difficult to understand. Why did the experts react as they did? For one thing, they were confident that they would turn out to be right. The tests are expensive and the experts receive a large share of the money paid for test fees. But, what is more important, they failed to see that their behavior had an impact on the welfare of patients.

Two studies, both poorly designed and carried out, concluded that the combination of ventilation and perfusion scanning was sufficiently accurate for the purpose of diagnosing pulmonary embolism. These studies were published in a journal devoted to nuclear medicine. The reviewers of these articles undoubtedly tried to be as fair and objective as possible, but to assign experts to judge themselves hardly constitutes a guarantee of objectivity.

In 1983, a well-designed prospective study from Canada essentially confirmed the findings of the 1977 analysis. The conclusions, although written in circumspect terms, were clear. Clinical evaluation of pulmonary embolism was unreliable: A negative perfusion scan ruled out the disease, but a positive perfusion scan was grossly unreliable. In most patients, the combination of the ventilation and perfusion scan resulted in major errors.

This study is as close to the truth as it is currently possible to come. If the Canadian study is valid, as seems likely, previous reports in the nuclear medicine literature were simply wrong. Currently, the National Heart, Lung, and Blood Institute of the National Institutes of Health is sponsoring an extensive study of these issues. The results are predictable; the National Heart, Lung, and Blood Institute's current extensive study will confirm the Canadian experience.

As the limitations of diagnosis by scanning have become progressively clearer, what has changed in patient care? Very little. Critics of the positive perfusion scan have won every battle, but patients continue to lose the war. Patient management is often still based on tests acknowledged to be inaccurate. The sad fact is that even after convincing evidence appears, doctors are painfully slow to translate it into patient management. Even after some doctors have learned that a practice is incorrect, they sometimes continue it. Others, because they are unaware of the issues, continue to practice as they always have.

Some three to five years down the line, results of the National Institutes of Health study will become available. Even assuming that these results unequivocally call attention to the inadequacies of scanning, major changes in practice may not take place for years.

The Pattern of Iatroepidemics

All three examples of iatroepidemics share several characteristics: A practice was introduced into medicine on the basis of a fundamentally unsound idea or poorly interpreted experience. The practice took hold without adequate studies to establish its efficacy and then developed a life of its own. It was supported by a group of experts whose opinions encouraged its continued use. Their own reputations or positions partially depended on the practice and, when challenged, they leaped to its defense. As a result, changes were slow to come. Because the idea was fundamentally unsound, many patients were harmed. This process, repeated time and again, fosters iatroepidemics.

To be thorough we should compare these three examples with another of a different order. Let's say a microbiologist has a good idea: Having found that a certain type of fungus kills bacteria, he uses an extract of that fungus to isolate the bacteria he is studying. A colleague suggests that the fungal extract can be used to treat a bacterial infection of the breast in cattle. This works, too. Then the idea is extended to the treatment of bacterial infections in humans. It is tried first in small groups of patients and then in a trial of extraordinary dimension. The world is at war and an organization exists for a trial of unprecedented magnitude—thousands of patients are tested and ultimately millions of lives are saved. This fungal extract was penicillin.

How can we determine which idea will lead to a medical triumph and which to an iatroepidemic? The answer is that only after preliminary studies on a broad enough scale can we establish benefits and risks. Without such trials, we are doomed to a certain number of iatroepidemics.

A Survey of Some Iatroepidemics

Before discussing iatroepidemics further, we should consider whether they are sporadic, rare events, or whether they are common. Following is a list of two dozen iatroepidemics with a brief description of each; the list is by no means complete. We should bear in mind that some of these iatroepidemics occurred before the importance of clinical trials was appreciated.

1. *Diethylstilbestrol (DES) to prevent spontaneous abortion.* The drug DES was administered to millions of pregnant women to

prevent abortion. It did not prevent abortion, but it did have another and unexpected effect: It exposed the children of the treated women to the development of genital cancer at relatively early ages.

2. *High oxygen exposure and blindness in children.* Although oxygen is known to be toxic to many tissues, numerous premature infants were treated with high oxygen concentrations without adequate precautions. The eyes of many were injured by a disease called retrolental fibroplasia. By the 1950s this disease was the leading cause of blindness in children. The irony is that the treatment with oxygen was unnecessary in most of the infants; there was no difference in survival between premature infants routinely treated with oxygen and those not treated.

There is now, in 1984, a new epidemic of retrolental fibroplasia. In my opinion, this epidemic results from two factors. One is that very premature infants now survive because of better care, and their retinas are probably more sensitive to the toxic effects of oxygen. The second is the introduction of new technologies that underestimate the levels of oxygen in the blood, which leads to the overuse of oxygen in these more susceptible infants.

3. *Biguanidines, associated with lactic acidosis.* Biguanidines, an oral drug used to treat diabetes, produced a life-threatening and sometimes fatal complication called lactic acidosis, a condition in which the blood becomes highly acidic, as a result of which the patient may die.

4. *Internal mammary artery ligation for coronary artery disease.* An artery in the chest is tied to increase blood supply to the heart. Designed to protect patients from heart attacks, this operation proved to be of no value. Before this was demonstrated, huge numbers of patients underwent the procedure and suffered pain, disability, and, occasionally, death.

5. *Exercise radionuclide ventriculograms for screening patients for coronary artery studies.* A test for selecting patients who might

benefit from invasive studies of the coronary arteries (blood vessels supplying the heart) was introduced. Studied on a small group, the test was found to be highly specific. Patients without coronary artery disease were said to have negative tests and patients with coronary artery disease to have positive tests. The test was and is widely used to select patients who ultimately go on to have coronary bypass surgery.

It was discovered that an elementary error had been committed in determining the specificity of the test—"studying the sickest of the sick and the wellest of the well." The original studies had used only normal people (the wellest of the well) and patients with far-advanced coronary artery disease (the sickest of the sick). This form of error is commonly overlooked in the attempt to establish the validity of various tests. Applied to a group of patients whose disease fell between the two extremes, it turned out to be no more specific than flipping a coin. As most patients fall between the two extremes, the test resulted in masses of patients undergoing an invasive procedure—coronary angiography—and, occasionally, bypass surgery. Past experience suggests that use of the test will persist for years, perhaps indefinitely, despite its obvious lack of specificity.

6. *Ileal bypass and obesity.* The last segment of the small intestine (the ileum) was bypassed by a surgical procedure to help patients lose weight. This procedure resulted in liver disease, arthritis, and even death in significant numbers of patients and has now been abandoned. Survivors still suffer from the complications of the surgery. Attempts to remove the bypass have created a second wave of complications.

7. *Chloramphenicol and bone marrow depression.* An antibiotic agent causes depression of the bone marrow, resulting in disability or death in some patients. In very specific circumstances the agent is uniquely suitable and even lifesaving. However, it is also used for trivial indications, when less toxic antibiotics could be used or when no antibiotics are necessary.

8. *Tonsillectomy in children.* For many decades, tonsillectomy was performed in millions of children on a more or less routine basis. In most cases, the operation was unnecessary. Some children were injured and some died (perhaps 1 in 10,000 or 15,000 operations) as a direct result of this largely unnecessary surgery. Evidence indicates that the removal of tonsils handicaps the body's defense mechanisms against infections. There are rare instances in which tonsillectomy is justified— for example, in some children the tonsils may obstruct breathing. Despite evidence that indicates no general benefit, tonsillectomy is the single most common surgical procedure in children. Some 400,000 are performed annually in the United States. Some tonsillectomies are used to treat children with a poorly described and diagnosed disease, glue ear.

9. *Psychosurgery for schizophrenia.* Several different brain operations were devised and performed on many mentally ill patients in the mistaken belief that surgery would improve their disease. The operations were not abandoned until thousands of patients were operated upon and many became even more disabled than before.

10. *Pneumothorax for tuberculosis.* Air was instilled in the pleural space (the space between the membranes covering the lung) in patients with pulmonary tuberculosis. In retrospect, the treatment not only was ineffective for tuberculosis but actually aggravated the disability.

11–12. *Adrenalectomy (surgical removal of the adrenal glands) and sympathectomy (removal of part of the nervous system) for high blood pressure.* These were two surgical procedures performed in order to treat high blood pressure. Adrenalectomy was done in relatively few patients; they did poorly. Sympathectomy was done in many patients; they either did not improve or became worse.

13–14. *Thyroid removal or thyroid suppression by drugs as treatment for coronary artery disease or chronic lung disease.* The thyroid gland was surgically removed or suppressed by drugs in order to decrease the oxygen requirements in patients with coronary artery disease or chronic lung disease. Before these approaches were abandoned, a large number of patients wound up with two separate diseases—their original disease and hypothyroidism (too little thyroid activity).

15. *Superficial femoral vein ligation for pulmonary embolism.* The superficial veins of the thigh were tied to prevent blood clots in leg veins from reaching the blood vessels of the lung. Blood clots from these veins did not pose a major danger of pulmonary embolism. In addition, many of the patients operated on did not have pulmonary embolism.

16. *Leukemia-causing agents for trivial or inappropriate diseases.* A number of patients were treated with very potent drugs (immunosuppressive drugs) which have as a late complication the development of leukemia. These agents were, for example, used in bronchial asthma and certain skin diseases that could have been controlled by less dangerous drugs.

17. *Flow-directed catheters in the blood vessels of the lung.* A catheter is floated into the blood vessels of the lung to measure the pressure in these blood vessels. This test is done in large numbers of critically ill patients, despite the fact that the measurements are of no real value in improving the treatment for most of these patients. Use of these catheters carries a small, but significant, incidence of complications. Occasionally, the complications cause death.

18. *Gastrojejunostomy for peptic ulcer.* In this operation for peptic ulcer (ulcer of the stomach or the first part of the small intestine), the stomach is joined to the midportion of the small intestine. After being performed in huge numbers of patients, it was found to be not particularly helpful.

19. *Subtotal gastrectomy for peptic ulcers.* A large part of the stomach was removed in patients with peptic ulcer. After surgery, patients frequently became malnourished and the long-term rate of complications was significant. The operation has been abandoned because it did little, if any, good.

20. *Thalidomide.* The thalidomide story is well known. This sedative drug taken by millions of women early in pregnancy caused an epidemic of children born with severely deformed limbs—6,000 to 8,000 cases in West Germany alone. It is of some interest that this drug now shows promise in the treatment of Behçet's syndrome—ulceration of the mouth and genitals, eye changes, and arthritis. The risk-benefit ratio of this drug will ultimately depend on the condition being treated.

21a. *Radiation for acne.* A high incidence of cancer of the skin occurred among patients who had earlier been treated by x-ray to the skin.

21b. *Radiation for status thymaticus.* Normal infants were considered to be at risk from enlargement of the thymus gland in the neck and many were treated prophylactically with x-ray to the neck. As a result, an unknown number developed cancer of the thyroid gland. It is now known that the disease never existed.

21c. *Radiation therapy for ankylosing spondylitis.* Radiation therapy to the spine was given to patients for a form of arthritis. The incidence of leukemia in these patients increased to tenfold that found in a controlled population. The incidence of cancer in the area that was radiated also increased to tenfold that found in controls.

22. *Hexachlorophene and brain damage in newborns.* An antiseptic agent (hexachlorophene or pHisoHex) with which nurses in nurseries for newborns scrubbed their hands was occasionally absorbed through the skin of premature infants, resulting in brain damage.

23. *Entero-Vioform and neurologic disease.* A new disease, characterized by visual impairment and degeneration of the spinal cord, appeared in Japan in the 1950s. Many of the more than 10,000 cases resulted in death. The disease was shown to be caused by the drug Entero-Vioform, prescribed for millions of Japanese patients for treatment of mild intestinal symptoms.

24. *Excess deaths in asthmatic children.* Inordinately high doses of a drug administered by inhalation caused a significant number of needless deaths in asthmatic children.

By no means all recognized iatroepidemics have been listed. Not all iatroepidemics are recognized. At any given time, most are hidden. Unless and until special circumstances arise, they remain unidentified.

Iatroepidemics and Medical Progress

We are in a period of rapid accumulation of new scientific knowledge and a corresponding increase in the introduction of new technologies, not all of which are good for patients. Without an organized system for detecting and eliminating iatroepidemics, the rapid expansion of information is inevitably accompanied by an increase in systematic errors. Depressing—and perhaps surprising—as the thought may be, patients are at a greater, not smaller, risk as medicine's scientific and technological base grows. This does not mean that the expansion of science and technology should be halted, but that we need to improve our approaches to the use we make of science and technology.

Many of the limitations of medicine that exist at any given time are due to unrecognizable and unforeseeable gaps in knowledge. With time, these gaps are filled and the limitations overcome. We know this random progression as medical progress. At times, the dividing line between a gap in medical progress and an iatroepidemic is blurred, but the distinction is real and significant.

An important characteristic of iatroepidemics is that they are not inevitable. At some point, the error that produced any of the epidemics listed could, or should, have been recognized and corrected. As an example of the distinction between an iatroepidemic and a gap in medical knowledge, consider the following: For many years patients with manic-depressive psychosis were treated by psychotherapy alone. Then lithium was found to be immeasurably more effective in many of these patients. This discovery could not have been anticipated, and to consider the previous psychiatric approaches to the disease as an iatroepidemic would be incorrect.

Identifying the Causes of Iatroepidemics

Even using the most generous criteria for judging our medical system, we can identify a host of systematic errors that cannot be considered inevitable consequences of the imperfect state of medical science. These errors are the root cause of iatroepidemics. We should ask about any systematic error in medicine: What was known? What should have been known? What should have been done? What can we say of those iatroepidemics taking place now or of those that will take place in the future? Industry faces similar responsibilities. For example, a number of diseases are caused by exposure to asbestos, a material used in industry. There is sometimes a long delay between exposure and development of asbestos-related disease. At what point should industry have taken steps to protect its workers by minimizing their exposure to asbestos? As soon as the danger became known, of course.

After the publication of Semmelweis's study, for example, obstetricians should have considered washing their hands prior to vaginal examinations. Surgeons should have conducted a careful comparison of radical mastectomy with less radical approaches in treating cancer of the breast after 1955. The nuclear medicine experts should have insisted on a careful evaluation of their techniques for diagnosing pulmonary embolism before introducing them for widespread use.

The distinction between a lag in medical progress and an iatroepidemic is not academic. Harm suffered because of inadequate medical knowledge is not predictable. An iatroepidemic is predictable and preventable.

Specialists and Generalists

Individual practicing physicians can do little about iatro-epidemics. Doctors must base their treatment on the best information available to them at the moment. They have no alternative; because their own knowledge and experience are necessarily limited they must depend on experts in various fields. When the experts are wrong, the patient suffers.

A serious dilemma for modern medicine is how to reconcile the role of medical specialists with that of medical generalists. Specialists focus on a narrow spectrum of diseases or a particular technique. They may know a great deal about their specialties but little about other aspects of medicine that affect patients' welfare. Some specialists have little or no direct relationship with patients. A specialist in diagnostic x-ray, for example, may know the patient only by his x-ray. A specialist in clinical pathology may know about a patient only what he learns by studying his laboratory tests. Generalists in medicine —general practitioners, family medicine practitioners—have a smattering of knowledge about many diseases, but often little in-depth knowledge or experience about many of the illnesses they treat.

In a real sense, modern medicine typifies the old aphorism that a specialist "learns more and more about less and less until he knows everything about nothing." A generalist, on the other hand, "learns less and less about more and more until he knows nothing about everything." Given this difference in emphasis, we cannot expect individual doctors to recognize, let alone do much about, iatroepidemics. Some other factors facilitate the development and perpetuation of iatroepidemics. Medical care is not a science and its practitioners are not scientists, although doctors may believe that they are acting from a scientific base as established in the medical literature. Most doctors do not recognize the tentative nature of medical "truth," let alone scientific "truth." When the medical literature is incorrect, patients suffer.

That medicine is not a science has some positive features: Physicians can be pragmatic in dealing with problems; they can be sympathetic toward the many patient complaints not susceptible to scientific analysis; they can, if they choose, reject a course of treatment recommended by established practice when they consider it not in the best interests of the patient; and they can act from humanistic and not scientific considerations.

The Importance of Clinical Trials

I have emphasized the need for clinical trials to determine the value of various diagnostic and therapeutic measures. The wrong questions, however, are too often incorporated into the design and interpretation of such studies. The only correct question to be posed is, Does a given approach improve the chances for survival or improve the life of the patient?

Two examples illustrate the point. You will recall that a published study measured the effect of long-term oxygen administration on the number of red cells in the blood of persistent smokers versus ex-smokers. The ex-smokers showed more nearly normal values than did the recalcitrant smokers. This was extrapolated to the conclusion that recalcitrant smokers do not respond to oxygen treatment and that it should therefore be withheld from them. Actually, the study did not determine whether long-term oxygen use was good for the smokers or not. This may lead to an iatroepidemic of withholding oxygen from patients who could benefit from its use and thereby harming them.

A recent study investigated whether the use of a particular catheter placed in the pulmonary blood vessels provided more accurate information about the patient than physical examination alone. The answer was that it did provide more accurate information. But to what end? Was the information of value in prolonging life or making possible a better life for the patients? This question was not asked. Based on present evidence, the most probable answer is no. Mortality rates in patients in whom the method is used are almost certainly not improved over those of ten years ago, when catheters were not widely used. But there is little doubt that the study, as published, will foster overuse of the the test. Moreover, both morbidity and mortality are associated with this particular test; an iatroepidemic may be in process.

Not only must it pose the right question, but the clinical trial, to be of value, must be a carefully controlled prospective trial (as explained in Chapter 2). *Controlled* refers to comparing untreated to treated subjects. In its simplest form, a controlled clinical trial is a study in which a group of patients are subjected to a given intervention and the results compared with those of a group not subjected to the intervention (the control group). *Prospective* refers to doing the study in a way agreed upon in advance and in an ongoing manner, that is, gathering the results as the study is done, as opposed to a retrospective study. The *retrospective* study depends upon medical records or information gathered in the past and not obtained under the rigorous conditions specified for evaluating the procedure being examined.

It is—and should be—difficult to enlist patients in these studies. (See Chapter 13 for a discussion of the patient as subject.) For the trial to be valid, closely matched groups of patients must be studied. This is not easy to achieve, as patients with the disease may have dissimilar hereditary, medical, and social backgrounds. Patients tend to react to the same alteration in diverse ways. This is called *biologic variation* and is an important factor in interpreting the results of clinical trials. The nature and stage of the disease in the patients under study should resemble the nature and stage of the disease in the population in which the invervention will ultimately be used. Otherwise, the results may not be applicable to the larger group.

Some Limitations of Clinical Trials

Another problem: If the treatment being tested seems effective, should the study be terminated and the control (untreated) group be given the benefit of the new treatment? It has happened that investigators have terminated a study prematurely because the results seemed favorable. As a result, the value of the particular intervention may never be known. For example, a study was performed to test the usefulness of an anticlotting agent, heparin, used in the treatment of blood clots in the lung. Heparin was used in half the patients and no heparin in the other half. During the study, three times as many deaths occurred in patients not on heparin as occurred in those taking the drug. The doctors terminated the study, considering it immoral to withhold an effective drug from any patient with a serious disease.

Unfortunately, the study had serious flaws. The number of patients studied was too small to justify the conclusions. Furthermore, it developed that a number of the patients did not have pulmonary embolism. The patients who died may have died of other diseases. No one has dared to repeat the study, and heparin is now given routinely to patients with a definite diagnosis of pulmonary embolism.

Would it have been unethical to continue the study so that firm conclusions could be drawn beyond the preliminary results indicating that the drug was effective? From the standpoint of hundreds of thousands of patients who have since received heparin without firm evidence of its effectiveness, certainly not. In point of fact, since that study was abandoned and no one since has repeated it, doctors do not know for certain that the treatment is helpful. A recent study suggests that heparin may not always be necessary in the treatment of pulmonary embolism. If so, its use will have constituted a major iatroepidemic because the drug can harm patients.

On the other hand, a clinical trial itself may pose a risk. Because of the length of time necessary to conduct the trial, the general introduction of a worthwhile treatment may be delayed, thereby harming groups of patients.

A poorly done clinical trial may produce what doctors call "the tomato effect." During the eighteenth century, tomatoes were cultivated and eaten in South America and Europe, but in North America there was a mistaken belief that tomatoes were poisonous and they were excluded from the diet. In medicine, the tomato effect refers to the unwarranted rejection of a highly efficacious therapy for unjustifiable reasons.

Other difficulties are inherent in these studies. Clinical trials are costly. As an area for research, they are not considered glamorous; exciting new ground is not broken. Long periods of time (sometimes years) may pass before the results of a clinical trial become available. Doctors may well be reluctant to undertake such long-term commitments, only, in some instances, to achieve results less clear-cut than required for guidance. Even with the best-designed trial, a simple black or white answer may not emerge. All these difficulties notwithstanding, adequate trials are probably the patients' best protection against being subjected to unwarranted risks.

The minutiae intrinsic to patient care are so numerous that it is doubtful that there would be sufficient time to study them all by clinical trials. There are, however, areas in which clinical trials are regularly pursued. New drugs proposed for human use must go through a fairly well-defined process before they can be introduced for treatment, as must new medical devices.

The need for an expansion of clinical trials is increasingly urgent as new drugs, instruments, tests, and technology are introduced into medical practice. As you may remember, a recent study indicated that more treatable diagnoses were missed by doctors in 1980 than in 1960, which suggests that the array of new gadgetry in modern medicine may not serve to improve the outcome for all patients.

The Development of Medical Knowledge

To understand how new iatroepidemics develop, one must know the basic process by which medical practices are incorporated into patient care. This process may be examined in three separate segments: *Transcription*—how the approach becomes inscribed in the minds of doctors; *translation*—how the approach is used in patient care; and *decay*—how the approach is found to be inadequate and modified or discarded.

Transcription

The introduction of new medical practices depends extensively on "the medical literature," which consists largely of medical journals. Incredibly numerous, they differ greatly in degree of sophistication, broadness of focus, and the intensity with which they scrutinize material submitted for publication.

Most commonly, an article submitted by an author is sent out for so-called peer review. One or two experts read the article, screen it for accuracy and relevance, and recommend its acceptance or rejection. The editor usually accepts the reviewers' recommendations. Inevitably, errors are made. Articles that might have a salutary influence on medical science are rejected, and articles that have an adverse influence are published. No one knows how common these episodes are, but there are stunning examples.

One of the most important scientific contributions of the twentieth century, a contribution that was to win the Nobel Prize for its author—the discovery of the process by which cells derive energy from foodstuff—was rejected by a famous journal, to be ultimately published in a less prestigious journal. The paper describing the use of a new test, radioimmunoassay, which has revolutionized some areas of medicine, after two unfavorable peer reviews, was rejected by the most prestigious medical science journal in the United States. This work was also awarded the Nobel Prize.

Conversely, an article claiming that bronchial asthma was caused by worms was published in a very famous medical journal. The claim was simply wrong. Another recent report associated worms with preeclampsia-eclampsia, a group of important diseases affecting pregnant women and manifested by high blood pressure, decreases in kidney function, and sometimes coma, convulsions, and death. Worms in the blood of these patients were identified and suggested as the cause of preeclampsia-eclampsia. So convinced were the investigators of the validity of their findings that they even named the worm —*Hydatoxi lualba*. Their evidence was that the injection of these worms into mice and dogs caused a disease similar to preeclampsia-eclampsia. Another group of investigators recently reassessed the findings and concluded that the "worms" were probably plant fibers and talc from surgical gloves worn by the investigators that had contaminated the blood samples that were being studied!

The original investigators were sufficiently principled to publicly acknowledge the findings of the second group of investigators. The point here is not that the original investigators made an error, but that the error was accepted as a reasonable approximation of the truth by several peer reviewers.

Fraud may be more difficult to detect than error. The inventor tends to be very persuasive when describing his fraudulent results. It happens only rarely (we hope) that articles are published by doctors who know that their results are fictitious. Although outright fraud is probably relatively uncommon in medicine, it does exist. Trivia and junk also find their way into the medical literature. It may well be that no system can be devised to upgrade the medical literature, but medicine should at least keep score. A computerized ongoing study could be developed to determine the effectiveness of the peer-review system in producing information with positive effects on patient care over a ten-year period. Using the computer to keep track of serious errors would also help.

Some of the medical literature is not subjected to peer review. Medical journals supported by advertisements paid for by drug companies and other commercial ventures often solicit from experts. In general, their requirements for accuracy are substantially less stringent and the articles tend to contain more "pearls"—opinions of the writer on various specific aspects of medical care.

A vast array of medical books and textbooks embraces every field of medicine. These combine a distillation of the medical literature with the personal opinions of, and interpretations by, the various authors. Post-graduate medical education is an extensively developed enterprise and assumes various forms —meetings, courses, special textbooks, video tapes among others.

Another source of information is the pharmaceutical company representative or "detail man" assigned to visit physicians in order to promote products. Along with information, he provides a supply of free drugs, much of which is donated to patients. When the drug is effective and safe, this serves a useful social purpose.

An interesting new method of establishing medical truths has recently emerged—the consensus conference. A group of experts in a specific, and usually controversial, area of medicine is assembled to consider pertinent issues and to come up with a series of recommendations—excellent idea, but it has shortcomings: The composition of the conference is determined by a chairman or committee, and too often the group is dominated by experts who have a personal stake in the outcome. A meeting, for example, called to consider a new form of treatment for blood clots was dominated by participants who had already endorsed the treatment. Not surprisingly, they enthusiastically reaffirmed their stance. The endorsement may turn out to be justified, but not by virtue of the objectivity of the meeting.

Again, the participants at a consensus conference called to discuss the value of intensive care units were almost exclusively doctors with high professional stakes in promoting these units. Many of the most pressing problems associated with intensive care units were not discussed, but the chairman summarized the deliberations by indicating that although no adequate data were available, it was clear that the units were of great value. How this conclusion was reached was not divulged.

From this vast array of amorphous material emerges what is considered to be the medical "truth" at any one time. This truth may not last very long, and may indeed be replaced by a truth completely at odds with it. Given the haphazard nature of medical knowledge, this startling shift may go unnoticed. It is hardly surprising that iatroepidemics can arise and flourish.

Many of the same imperfections are found in science, but there is a difference. In science, these imperfections lead to intellectual errors; in medicine, they harm human beings directly.

Translation

The process by which physicians translate material into practice has little rhyme or reason.

At a meeting of gastrointestinal specialists, the question was asked, How many of you believe that ——— [a drug] is useful in treatment of gastrointestinal hemorrhage? Not a single hand was raised. The next question was, How many of you use this drug in the treatment of gastrointestinal hemorrhage? Approximately 99 percent of the specialists acknowledged that they did.

Sometimes doctors simply fail to act on information that is readily understood. They also commonly make interpretive errors. For example, a certain test in the literature is said to be accurate only when the chest x-ray of the patient is normal, but doctors use the test whether or not the chest x-ray is normal. A given form of treatment is said to be effective only in males; the treatment is used indiscriminately in both males and females.

Distortions can be individual or systematic. A patient was subjected to an extensive series of studies in order to determine whether she had an infection of the perirenal space

(space surrounding the kidney) or direct infection of the kidney itself. Her doctors justified the tests by quoting the medical literature to the effect that each of the two different kinds of infection required entirely different forms of treatment. The medical literature was reviewed and found to state the exact opposite—the treatment for the two conditions was identical. Doctors, like other human beings, can misunderstand the printed word.

Decay

When new tests or treatments are described, the results are quickly transmitted to the medical community, but the process of the decay of poor practices may be inordinately slow, although there have been some notable exceptions.

Some delay is the result of cultural lag. By the time the originators of a method, in Boston for example, decide to withdraw their proposal, doctors 2,000 miles away may be just introducing it. And there is a reluctance to admit mistakes. Because peer pressure operates strongly to punish the doctor responsible for introducing or supporting a bad method, errors are not commonly acknowledged. Again, there are notable exceptions. Medical journals dislike publishing retractions, because these are usually considered to be of little interest. Without an organized vehicle for publishing errors and an organized basis for discovering systematic errors, many iatroepidemics go undetected, and the lessons that could be derived from studying them are almost never widely disseminated, so that the process of decay is prolonged.

The nature of medical school training also inhibits the decay of harmful medical practices. Too little attention is given to helping the student learn what *not* to do and when not to do it. No structural approach to the critical evaluation of the medical literature is provided and the hazards of overusing technology are not emphasized. There is no place in the curriculum for systematic analysis of iatrogenic episodes and iatroepidemics. Arrogance tends to dull perception, so that errors are either not recognized, or not acknowledged and eliminated. Humility tends to be in short supply among both students and faculty in most medical schools. The atmosphere of the school does not suggest its importance, and humility is a quality difficult to teach in formal courses.

Preventing Iatroepidemics

Iatroepidemics cannot be directly controlled by individual doctors, but for medicine as a whole there are some effective measures: First, to openly acknowledge the existence of iatroepidemics; once a problem is acknowledged, solutions can emerge. Then, to expand the use of improved clinical trials—major support for these would almost certainly have to originate with the government—coupled with a surveillance system to monitor and expose incipient iatroepidemics.

If peer pressure operated to encourage frank acknowledgment of honest mistakes, it would become more respectable to admit errors quickly. Medicine should take responsibility for organizing something like an *International Journal of Errors, Amendments, and Retractions.* The authors would be physicians who had themselves published material they later found to be erroneous and experts who would analyze important errors made by others. This would permit many doctors, instead of a few, to learn from their own and others' errors.

Medicine has an antiquated, largely unstructured, and inadequate system for evaluating the flood of new approaches that are fast being introduced. Unless improvements are made in the system, iatroepidemics can be expected to increase sharply.

Perhaps the most effective single step would be to modify the curriculum of medical schools. Turning out young doctors who would use medicine to improve patient welfare directly, who were sharply aware of their own limitations and the limitations of medicine, who knew how to separate the wheat from the chaff, who could critically evaluate medical literature, who did not feel constrained to hide or suppress mistakes in patient care, would go a long way toward the eradication of iatro-epidemics.

9

Surgery: Necessary, Unnecessary, and In-Between

Thanks to the extraordinary advances in surgical technique over the past 20 years, the number of operations performed has vastly increased. Almost any patient is now a potential candidate for surgery, including many once judged too ill or too old to survive an operation. This has added a new risk—the risk of prolonging the survival of patients who may have no real hope of leading a useful or happy life after surgery. The risk-benefit analysis is accordingly more difficult.

Surgery has done no better than medicine as a whole in compiling or using data for careful risk-benefit analysis, and surgeons have little training for this new dimension of their practice. At present their technical competence may be outrunning their ability to make balanced decisions; one result has been the creation of a population of patients who, having survived surgery, are waiting to die. As the options increase, the need for the patient to accept responsibility for sharing in surgical decisions becomes more urgent.

Categories of Surgery

Surgeons have traditionally divided surgery into two categories: *Emergency surgery,* meaning that the surgery must be done immediately or the patient will die, and *elective surgery,* meaning either that the surgery is required but can be deferred until another time—"Mrs. Jones, your gall-bladder should come out but it does not have to be removed immediately"—or that the surgery is purely discretionary on the part of the patient. A face-lift would fall into this category.

A more useful classification for patients would subdivide surgery into three categories:

- *Necessary surgery,* meaning that the risk-benefit analysis indicates that the operation is likely to improve the patient's chances for a happy or productive life.
- *Unnecessary surgery,* meaning that the risk-benefit analysis indicates that the surgery is not likely to achieve that goal.
- *In-between surgery,* meaning that it is difficult to decide whether surgery is likely to help. In-between decisions are often resolved by operating. They might better be resolved by waiting and observing the course of the patient's illness.

You (and your surgeon) should remember an important principle: If surgery is postponed the chances are that it can, if necessary, be performed in the future. Once surgery is performed, the results are not reversible. This principle was graphically expressed by the great Russian writer Solzhenitsyn: "Any fool can cut a head off. It takes a magician to put one back." (For head substitute gallbladder, uterus, ovary, intestine.)

Necessary Surgery

In general we think of emergency surgery as necessary surgery, but that is an inaccurate definition. What is necessary for one patient may be unnecessary for another. Definition depends on the patient's view of a happy and productive life. For some patients, a face-lift or a mammaplasty (plastic reconstruction of the breast) is necessary surgery. The right to decide on surgery, as on any aspect of medical care, is the patient's, but it should be a choice informed by an explicit awareness of the risks.

Unnecessary Surgery

The information you need in order to distinguish between necessary and unnecessary surgery may not always be available, but you should know how extremely distorted the decision-making process of surgical experts can sometimes be. In this respect, the following story is instructive.

"Elective" Hysterectomy

In 1969, a respectable gynecological journal printed an editorial on "elective hysterectomy," proposing that the uterus should be removed surgically in (essentially) every woman past childbearing age, say, 35. "Elective" in the context of the editorial meant that there were no clear medical indications for the surgery. The basis of this modest proposal was summarized as follows:

> The uterus has but one function: Reproduction. After the last planned pregnancy, the uterus becomes a useless, bleeding, symptom-producing, potentially cancer-bearing organ and therefore should be removed.

The article further suggested:

> If, in addition, both ovaries are removed, further benefits occur. Replacement therapy [the prescribing of female sex hormones] is simple and inexpensive. Premenstrual tension is no longer a problem. Another source of inoperable malignancy is eliminated.

In accordance with medical tradition, a list of benefits was provided. No risks were considered.

1. The nuisance, inconvenience, and disability of menstrual periods are eliminated.

2. Pain and discomfort associated with menstruation are no longer a problem.

3. As it is a sterilizing operation, the need for prolonged use of contraceptives no longer exists. Fear of pregnancy is no longer disturbing. The tragedy of an unwanted pregnancy late in the menstrual life is eliminated.

4. Hospitalization for curettage and conization of the cervix, usually prepared for the purpose of biopsy, is no longer necessary.

5. There is no longer a need for the annual cytologic smear.

6. Fear of cancer of the uterus is eliminated; loss of life from cancer of this organ is now of no concern.*

Gynecologists were urged to show careful adherence to rules, to perform a careful workup, and to conform to prescribed regulations and procedures, but "after this careful evaluation, the gynecologist himself must make this decision." One might have thought that the patient would be the person to decide.

Was this a serious proposal? Indeed it was, and two years later (1971) the value of elective hysterectomy was debated at a meeting of the American College of Obstetrics and Gynecology. The proponents outclapped the opponents by a substantial margin, or at least, as recorded by an audiometer, more noisily. That a majority of the doctors at the meeting applauded the proposal cannot, however, be extrapolated to mean that a majority actually supported elective hysterectomy. The applause may have only been a judgment of relative debating skills and not of the merits of the underlying proposal.

The impact of the proposal on the number of hysterecto-

*Reprinted with permission from The American College of Obstetricians and Gynecologists. Ralph C. Wright, "Hysterectomy: Past, Present, and Future," *Obstetrics and Gynecology,* vol. 33, no. 4 (April 1969): 560.

mies performed in the United States has not been measured. Doctors who supported elective hysterectomy presumably would have performed some elective operations. Doctors who opposed elective hysterectomy, when confronted with in-between decisions—whether or not to perform hysterectomy when indications were borderline—would be more disposed to go ahead with the surgery. The conditions were thus set for a substantial increase in the number of hysterectomies performed. As quantitative data are not available, we cannot label the episode as an iatroepidemic, but it is probable that it initiated an epidemic of unnecessary hysterectomies, of which we have not seen the end.

How seriously doctors regarded the proposal may be judged by an article that appeared in 1976 in a prestigious medical journal. The article analyzed the pros and cons of elective hysterectomy and considered some of the risks, emphasizing the deaths and complications caused by hysterectomy. Data indicated that about 2 women per 1,000 hysterectomies died and about 350 per 1,000 suffered complications.

The analysis then took a tangential track, pointing out that women undergoing hysterectomy at age 35 have a longer life expectancy (42.1 years) than those who do not have the operation (41.9 years). One million hysterectomies would result in a total gain of 181,915 woman-years. Sounds impressive, does it not? The analysis largely ignored one important consideration—that perioperative deaths (deaths occurring as a result of complications surrounding the period of operation) occur quickly. Also, the problems that the surgery was supposed to prevent occur over many years. If a patient died of surgery at age 35 she would lose 40 years of life. If she survived to age 50 before dying of some form of uterine cancer, she would have lost only 25 years of life. Therefore, many more woman-years would be lost than gained by the operation.

The article estimated that proposed hysterectomies would cause 600 deaths in women aged 35. The estimate did not include women of 40, 50, and 60 years of age, although they would also be provided the "benefits" of elective hysterectomy. Including all women over the age of 35 in the proposal would take a staggering toll. Assuming that 75 million women are in those age groups, most of American life would rotate around the performance of hysterectomies. This would cause a minimum of 150,000 deaths in normal women, and 25 million normal women, or one-third the total, would have iatrogenic complications.

The authors of the article based their conclusions on two sweeping but flimsy assumptions. One, that the difference between 42.1 years and 41.9 years represented a *significant* difference in survival. This actually amounts to 0.2 years, or one-fifth of a year, or 73 days. Two, that if this difference were truly significant it could be attributed to a single factor—whether or not the patient had a hysterectomy. If you were a doctor reading this expert analysis, especially if you already had a bias toward elective hysterectomy, this part of the analysis would support your prejudice.

The article finally concluded that universal elective hysterectomy was probably unwarranted, not because it might do harm, but because to do the required number would cost too much money and consume too many resources. This is a classic example of a correct conclusion arrived at for mostly the wrong reasons: "The idea was good, it just cost too much."

In the past six years, the concept of universal elective hysterectomy seems to have faded away, for reasons that are not clear. The rate at which hysterectomies are performed, however, still reflects this concept.

We can see from this episode how easy it may be for doctors to perform great numbers of unnecessary operations. We can also see the process by which a potentially harmful medical practice becomes ingrained in medicine. Table 9-1 shows the process: Some doctor or group of doctors has what amounts to a harebrained or poor idea. He or they provide a convincing rationale. Although the potential benefits are emphasized

Table 9-1

Steps in the Development of Bad Medical Practices

1. A bad idea.	An aging uterus is useless and can cause trouble. Take it out.
2. Inadequate analysis.	Benefits of hysterectomy are considered. Risks are largely ignored.
3. Many doctors are convinced by the analysis.	Medical literature and postgraduate meetings disseminate the idea of elective hysterectomies.
4. The idea is implemented and used on many patients without an adequate data base.	Elective hysterectomy and in-between hysterectomies increase. It would have been impossible to test elective hysterectomies by a clinical trial, and the idea should have been abandoned before it was used on patients.
5. Theoretical analyses of the idea are complex and fail to identify the major problems. The criticisms are so vague, fuzzy, and polite that they convince few physicians.	The tentative conclusion by public health experts is that elective hysterectomy probably saves woman-years but costs too much.
6. The practice is widely used, ultimately fading away for reasons that are not clear.	There was never a formal repudiation of elective hysterectomy.

and the potential risks overlooked, many doctors are convinced, and a large number of patients are subjected to a procedure whose value has not been established by adequate studies.

Ultimately criticisms are leveled at the practice, usually on theoretical rather than factual grounds. Even when they are negative, they are often so obscurely stated that they fail to persuade doctors who have accepted the original proposal. Even without public acknowledgment, however, doctors usually abandon the grossest errors; the practice fades away, leaving a trail of usually unrecognized victims.

Elective hysterectomy raises a key point not discussed before: Some important proposals cannot be tested by clinical trials. It would have been impossible to select three groups of 35-year-old women and subject one-third of them to hysterectomy, one-third to a sham hysterectomy (the abdomen would be opened but uterus and ovaries not removed), and leave one-third unaltered. The very idea of such a study curdles the blood. Any practice affecting the welfare of thousands of patients should not be introduced if it cannot be tested by a clinical trial.

Surgery in Normal Breasts

The uterus is not the only organ recommended for removal while still apparently healthy. In women who develop cancer of one breast, some doctors urge the removal of the apparently normal remaining breast. They reason that a woman with cancer of one breast is at risk of developing cancer of the remaining breast. The risk is said to be greater than 10 percent; estimates are that this is a greater risk than that associated with surgical removal. Some studies suggest that in many patients, perhaps most patients, the apparently normal breast does contain some cancer cells. In the overwhelming number of patients, however, these cells do not go on to multiply and to produce clinically important cancer.

Again, the only way to justify removing an apparently normal breast would be to perform a clinical trial that would compare the outcome in patients with bilateral breast removal with that in patients who had removal of only the diseased breast. Such a study would be most difficult to conduct, and therefore we have no adequate data to support or refute the value of removing the apparently normal breast. This does not stop some surgeons. Women with fibrocystic disease (a number of cysts in both breasts whose cause is not known) have had both breasts removed because it was believed that fibro-cystic disease was a precancerous lesion—an almost certainly incorrect assumption; most forms of fibrocystic disease are not precancerous.

In-Between Surgery

Mr. Bottle (name mythical, incident real) is 84 years old, hale and vigorous. He has a family history of polyps (small tumors) protruding in the large intestine, some of which may become cancerous. As a result, Mr. Bottle has frequent exami-nations of the inside of his large bowel by sigmoidoscopy. During one examination, a polyp was found and biopsied.

The first pathologist pronounced it a definite cancer and a surgeon urged removal of part of the large intestine. A second pathologist judged it to be a cancer in situ (nests of cancer cells in a localized area which had not spread). A second surgeon advised against an operation, and the original pathologist who had thought the polyp was invasive cancer now agreed that the second biopsy showed a cancer in situ. Several surgeons agreed that the large intestine should be spared but advised periodic sigmoidoscopic examinations.

Some months later the polyp, still there, was again biopsied; and this time both pathologists interpreted it as invasive can-cer. The original surgeon leaned toward no surgery; the sec-ond surgeon leaned toward surgery. They had exactly re-versed their positions. After much agonizing, everyone agreed that the decision was up to the patient himself. The main risk in rejecting surgery was that the cancer would ulti-mately cause his death; the benefit was that he would avoid the possibility of cutting short his remaining effective span of life. Moreover, surgery would disable him at least temporarily. He finally decided that he would not undergo surgery. The "cor-rect" decision is too close to call. In truth, there is none. The emotional trauma that this patient suffered stemmed from life and not from the actions of his doctors. This kind of vexing problem has to be considered case by case.

How Much Unnecessary Surgery Is Performed?

We can more profitably consider unnecessary surgery as a class of surgery. We have only indirect evidence that unnecessary surgery is common, but that evidence is compelling enough to alert potential patients to the risk of "oversurgery." Some of the evidence comes from Canada, where these issues are more actively studied than they are in the United States, and some comes from the United States. As practices appear to be quite similar in the two countries, information from both sources can be pooled.

Both Canada and the United States have surgical rates per unit of population approximately double those of Great Britain. This could mean that there is too little surgery in Great Britain, but, judging by death rate, age of survival, and general health of the population, this does not appear to be the case. These values are the same in Great Britain and in North America. Judging by data from Canada for 1968, the rates of elective surgery, such as hernia repair and hemorrhoidectomy, were especially high in Canada as compared with Great Britain. Radical mastectomy was 3.2 times greater in Canada, and hysterectomy more than twice as great. The death rates from cancer of the breast, cancer of the cervix, and cancer of the uterus were the same in both countries.

A comparison of the rate of surgery in the United States and Great Britain appears to reflect the number of surgeons per unit population. In 1970, there were twice as many surgeons per capita in the United States and twice as much surgery. One might conclude that the number of surgeons in Great Britain is inadequate, but this does not appear to be the case. On the contrary, almost every careful survey indicates that the United

States has an excessive supply of surgeons; furthermore, the surplus is increasing. True, in Great Britain elective surgery is less routinely available than in the United States. But this does not appear to have an adverse effect on survival and general health in Great Britain.*

Evidence of substantial amounts of unnecessary surgery includes the existence of surgical fads—operations that come and then go because they were poorly conceived or dangerous. Tonsillectomy, internal mammary ligation, elective hysterectomy, and ileal bypass are examples (see Chapter 8). What surgical fads of today will fade away tomorrow?

The Effect of Physicians' Strikes on Death Rates

Indirect evidence of unnecessary surgery is provided by an interesting and unexplained phenomenon: Death seems to take a partial holiday during doctors' strikes, when only emergency surgery is performed. Decreases in total death rate have coincided with such strikes in Canada, Israel, and Southern California. During each strike the total death rate decreased, but rose to its prestrike level after elective surgery was resumed.

To be fair, we must recognize that multiple factors undoubtedly contribute to this unusual but recurring phenomenon. To attribute the drop in death rate solely to the postponement of elective surgery would be to assume that the usual rate of death from elective surgery is high enough to affect the overall death rate significantly. This staggering assumption would lead to an even more staggering idea: If the services of all doctors were restricted to the minimum required for emer-

---

*There is a long wait for some forms of elective surgery in Great Britain. A patient may have to wait five years for the replacement of a hip. This may be bad for the quality of his life, but does not detract from the major conclusion. It has been suggested that surgery has little impact on public health statistics but primarily affects the quality of individual lives. There are no acceptable studies to validate this assumption.

gency care, would the death rate decline rather than rise? This is an old idea ingrained in American folklore, as this story bears witness: A surgeon stopped by at a general store. "Morning, Doc," said the owner, "where have you been?" "Oh, I was down south hunting." "Kill anything?" "Not a thing," said the doctor. "That's too bad," said the store-keeper. "You could have done better if you had stayed home and practiced your trade." The association between the physicians' strikes and the decreased death rate may be happenstance, but certainly deserves additional study.

Some Reasons Behind Unnecessary Surgery

If we assume that there is systematic overuse of surgery, can we identify its causes? One cause we have already mentioned: There are too many surgeons. Evidence shows that the amount of surgery increases as the number of surgeons increases. An increase in the frequency of surgery also appears to accompany an increase in surgical facilities. The fee-for-service system, which allows the doctor to set his own fee, has also been suggested as a possible factor, as it creates a sharp economic incentive for doing more surgery. This may well be true, but direct analysis of economic influences is complex.

The nature of our medical care system and of medical training plays a role here as it does in other aspects of medicine. Surgeons, like other doctors, are trained to "do their thing." Their thing is operating. Critical assessment of what not to do and when not to do it is too little emphasized in their training. Most standard textbooks of surgery, for example, do not mention the death rate associated with various surgical procedures and some do not mention the rates of complication. One would suppose this information to be critical, and some of it is available in the medical journals. However, sometimes when surgeons are questioned about the morbidity and mortality of specific procedures, they do not know.

Avoiding Unnecessary Surgery

It would be difficult to convince Mr. Lake (name mythical, incidents real) that unnecessary surgery is not rampant. When he developed a swelling of the parotid gland—a salivary gland in the cheek—surgery was advised. A second doctor dissented, believing that the swelling was probably an infection and not a tumor. He convinced Mr. Lake that even if the swelling was a tumor, he could afford to wait. He did and the swelling subsided.

Mr. Lake's best friend showed an abnormality of the lung on a chest x-ray and was advised to have a lung biopsy because of the possibility of cancer of the lung. He rejected the advice, and with antibiotic treatment the abnormality disappeared from the x-ray. While this was going on, a swelling of the thyroid gland was discovered in the same friend. One doctor advised a surgical biopsy of the thyroid gland to be followed by its removal if a cancer was present. Another doctor inserted a needle into the gland and found no cancer. The swelling receded with the passage of time and simple medication.

Mr. Lake's secretary was advised to have a hysterectomy because of an enlarged ovary detected in a physical examination. Mr. Lake insisted that she see another doctor. The second doctor found no enlarged ovary and no surgery was performed. Mr. Lake's daughter-in-law-to-be underwent an ultrasound examination of her abdomen as part of a "routine" premarital examination. The test detected an enlarged ovary and surgery was advised. When the original ultrasound examination was reinterpreted at another institution and the test repeated, the original test turned out to be a false positive. The first expert was misled by a normal fold of her large bowel, which he interpreted as an ovary. No surgery was necessary.

Minimizing the Risks of Surgery

Emergency or immediate life-saving surgery follows its own rules. If a patient with a bullet in the chest is hemorrhaging uncontrollably, surgery is mandatory. By definition, you have no alternative and must go ahead, whatever the circumstances and whatever the level of surgical skills and surgical competence and resources available to you.

When faced with elective surgery, be as sure as you can that the proposed operation will contribute to your well-being. Remember that unnecessary surgery is common. This means that you must insist that the surgeon extensively define his reasons for recommending surgery and predict the result he expects. Even if this insistence makes him impatient or uncomfortable, persevere. If he remains uncomfortable, find another surgeon.

The Second Opinion and Beyond

One precaution is to obtain a second opinion. The theory is that, if the two doctors concur, the chances are that the indications for surgery are valid. This is probably true in many circumstances, but remember that most practitioners will concur in a systematic error. Second opinions, for example, would not have prevented unnecessary tonsillectomies or hysterectomies. However, a second doctor may provide you with an opportunity to learn more about the risks and benefits of the proposed surgery so that you can make a more rational choice.

What if the two opinions differ? It may not be economically practical to get a third opinion. Moreover, which opinion should you accept? Is two out of three better than one out of two?

However many surgical opinions you obtain, you would be well advised to have a nonsurgical doctor as a major advisor.

This doctor's objective should be to help you reach the best decision possible. He should not be a surgeon for two reasons: He can provide a different kind of input, and he will have no stake in your decision to undergo or to reject surgery. He should be a doctor who enjoys your confidence and who is able to communicate with you. He can help you select the best place to go for surgery and the best available surgeon.

He would be your ombudsdoctor; his function will be discussed in a later chapter. As a representative and advocate of the patient, he would have no conflict of interest, would be able to explain the medical issues involved, and would help the patient make the most rational decision.

In most cases, your best option would be to follow the most cautious opinion. If the surgery is elective, postponing it as long as possible makes sense. This does expose you to certain risks. Postponing the removal of a gallbladder may result in emergency surgery under less favorable circumstances, but on balance is probably the lesser risk. Remember: Once surgery is performed, it cannot be unperformed. There is almost no such thing as a minor operation. (A minor operation is one that is performed on someone else.) Remember also that anesthesia alone can cause complications and death. By remembering these facts you will be inclined to be less passive and more involved in deciding whether or not to have surgery.

To minimize your risks you must be informed about all phases of your surgical care. The process of surgery can be divided into three segments. The risks of each segment, and the skills and resources required for each, are different. First is the preoperative period. Here diagnostic expertise, judgment, and skill in preparing the patient for surgery are key. In some instances, these tasks are delegated to others. The second segment is the operation itself. Here the technical skills of the surgeon and the surgical team are decisive; judgment and operating-room resources are also important. Third is the postoperative period. Many of the complications and deaths associated with surgery occur during this phase; busy surgeons frequently give insufficient attention to patients immediately after surgery. Postoperative care has significantly improved, in large measure because a skilled group of nurses is now available; they can make the difference between life and death. The postoperative period nevertheless remains a time of increased risk.

Try to have your surgery at the best place that is available and by the best surgeon you can find. Not all surgeons are equally competent and experienced in all areas. The resources and experience of one hospital may be substantially better than those of another. Morbidity and mortality differ markedly from one institution to another. This information is not easy to obtain and the choice demands a subjective judgment on your part. You (or your ombudsdoctor) can ask about the extent of your surgeon's experience and the record of the hospital with respect to surgery in general and your proposed operation in particular. You will also want to know about the adequacy of all three segments of surgery at the specific institution—preoperative, operative, and postoperative.

An ombudsdoctor would be particularly helpful to potential surgical patients. The pattern of referral for surgery commonly follows what has been called the "buddy" system. The surgeon who is recommended has close professional, economic, or personal ties to the referring physician. These are not acceptable criteria for selecting the most competent surgeon.

It is estimated that one-third of operations are still performed by doctors who have had no formal surgical training. An unknown number are performed by trained surgeons who failed to pass the qualifying examinations required to certify competence as a surgeon.

All of this can be summarized by saying that you must not be a silent or passive partner in a surgical experience. As a patient you have the largest stake in the outcome. You should therefore be aware of the important details that contribute to the decision whether to operate, when to operate, and where to operate.

10

The Critically Ill and the Not-So-Critically Ill

Hospital care of the critically ill has been revolutionized during the past 20 years. Its facilities for performing various measurements and for exhaustively monitoring patients increased the appeal of the intensive care unit (ICU), and as an organizational form it swept through the United States to become the center of hospital life.

Industry has responded by developing a variety of gadgets to monitor, measure, and treat ICU patients. More and more patients are admitted. Medical students and residents flock to be trained, attracted by the challenge, the excitement, the technology, and the appeal of making life-or-death decisions. Such decisions are made hurriedly, without much time for reflection, and usually in an aggressive fashion. When the stakes are life or death, it is considered acceptable to employ virtually any form of treatment that might help the patient. Much of routine care seems dull by comparison.

The Intensive Care Unit (ICU)

The ICU is a specially designated, geographically separate area of the hospital, staffed by a special team of physicians and a special team of nurses, and housing specialized equipment for monitoring and treating the critically ill.

These patients tend to have certain problems in common. They include:

- Respiratory failure—an inability of the lungs to absorb adequate amounts of oxygen and to excrete adequate amounts of carbon dioxide. These abnormalities are treated by using a ventilator, by supplying extra oxygen to the patient, and by other special measures designed to improve the function of the lung.
- Cardiovascular failure—insufficient oxygen is supplied to the tissues and insufficient carbon dioxide is removed; inadequate amounts of nutrients are supplied to the tissues and inadequate amounts of various toxic products are removed because the heart or blood vessels function abnormally. These abnormalities are treated by various measures designed to increase the effectiveness of the heart and to decrease the amount of work that the heart must perform and to improve blood vessel function.
- Renal failure—inability of the kidneys to adequately conserve various substances needed by the body and to excrete various waste products whose accumulation leads to dire consequences. This abnormality is treated by proper fluid administration and by dialysis (removal of various substances from the blood by a kidney machine or other techniques).
- Deficient clotting of the blood, leading to poorly controlled bleeding.
- Abnormalities of other organs, such as the brain and liver, which are sometimes related to the above problems.
- A high incidence of infection. Critically ill patients tend to be infected more easily than normal subjects. In some instances infection is actually the cause of the above abnormalities.

In view of the similarity of their illnesses and their needs, it seemed reasonable to keep all critically ill patients in a common facility, where a number of the devices and techniques necessary for treatment would be immediately available.

When patients are critically ill, it would seem important to measure various vital functions: The amount of oxygen and carbon dioxide in the blood, the blood pressure, the cardiac output (the amount of blood that the heart pumps each minute), and the amount of urine excreted per hour. The ability to measure and monitor a patient makes doctors feel they can really determine what is going on in that patient—whether or not they can act on the changes they observe. With the rapid development of new measuring techniques, the number of body functions that could be measured increased. Monitoring methods also increasingly depended upon complicated and costly equipment, all of which could be most efficiently housed in a single place.

Because the care of the critically ill is so demanding, it seemed useful to assemble a team of specially trained doctors. As time progressed, this idea took hold, and recently *critical-care medicine*—its practitioners are known as *intensivists*—has been formally recognized as a specialty within medicine.

These patients require unusually skilled and complex nursing care, and critical-care nurses are specially trained to provide such care. It can be and has been argued that the most valuable element of ICU care is the devotion and proficiency of the nurses, rather than the special technologies or skills of the doctors. (This can be explained, at least in part, by the favorable nurse-patient ratio. At any one time, a nurse looks after many fewer patients than a doctor does.)

Once the common elements in critical care were identified, various subgroups of ICUs developed. Surgical ICUs were organized for surgical patients, medical ICUs for medical patients, neonatal ICUs for the newborn, and pediatric ICUs for children. Some hospitals are not blessed with critical care specialists and, in such institutions, each physician cares for his own critically ill patient in a common facility.

At this point, you can predict the flaw: ICUs caught on and flourished without any careful clinical trials to establish their overall effectiveness. Do they, in fact, contribute to the chances for a happy and productive life for patients? The practice has been to try it on patients first and then, perhaps later—or never—to determine its effectiveness.

Who Benefits from the ICU?

For selected groups of patients the effectiveness of the ICU has either been demonstrated or can be inferred.

- Neonatal ICUs have been shown to improve the survival rate of premature infants significantly. These infants usually have well-circumscribed medical problems, and tiding them over a specific problem permits normal growth and development to occur.
- Patients suffering from an overdose of drugs, particularly drugs that depress breathing or injure the lungs, also appear to benefit from the ICU.
- Victims of accidents and other forms of trauma may benefit, because many of these are young people without previous disease.
- Patients with various forms of neurologic disease may also benefit, because, except for the neurologic disease, many are relatively normal.

Except for these groups, there is no acceptable evidence that care in the ICU improves more lives than it harms. In general, the risks of ICU admission have not been carefully analyzed, but some can be identified by considering the composition of the ICU patient population.

Is the ICU the Place for the Terminally Ill?

The terminally ill are often admitted to the ICU despite the fact that they have incurable diseases and will almost certainly die soon. They are admitted, literally, for the purpose of prolonging the process of their dying, rather than for the purpose of prolonging their lives. The risk is not that they will die but that they may die under needlessly painful circumstances. Is the ICU a suitable place for a dying patient to spend what little time remains? Most would agree that it is not. To spend the remaining hours of life hooked to a breathing machine, with tubes inserted into one's body orifices, and undergoing painful or uncomfortable, undignified tests and treatment, none of which can help, is surely a terrible way to die.

How great a portion of the ICU population do the terminally ill comprise? This varies from unit to unit. In a study conducted by one world-famous surgical ICU, 54 percent of patients admitted had died within a month; 75 percent had died within a year. Not all of the patients who died were terminal. Indeed, some of the group were most probably salvageable* and might have been saved but for incidental factors. Some of the group died almost certainly as a result of complications that developed during treatment. But the death rate was so high that it is safe to conclude that many terminally ill patients were admitted and died a needlessly uncomfortable, undignified death.

Identifying the Terminally Ill

The issues involved in deciding whether or not to admit terminal patients to an ICU are extraordinarily complex. To identify terminal illness is not always easy, especially in the early stages of a patient's hospital course, when little may be known about his medical problems and prognosis. It goes

---

*"Salvageable" is a blunt term widely used to describe patients who can be returned to a happy and productive life.

without saying that, if any doubt exists, the patient should be treated as vigorously as seems necessary. But terrible mistakes can be made.

A young man of 19 suffered from muscular dystrophy, a congenital disease characterized by weakness of the skeletal muscles, including those used for breathing. He developed a respiratory infection, and his breathing became progressively more difficult. His physician, a pediatric orthopedic surgeon who had taken care of him since childhood, asked that he be admitted to the adult ICU.

Some jurisdictional problems developed. The ICU doctors felt that the patient was not an appropriate admission for the ICU. Even before they had examined him, they concluded that he had an irreversible disease, which was true, and that he was not salvageable, which turned out to be false. The patient was admitted with considerable reluctance—the ICU doctors felt he had been "dumped" on them.

Physicians in ICUs work under terrible pressures. Required to make frequent and fateful decisions, they may respond by becoming arrogant. They often adopt a siege mentality—it's us against them ("they" are the non-ICU doctors "who don't know what they're doing"). ICU doctors work long hours and are subject to extreme fatigue. Typically, they tend to burn out after a number of years, and go on to practice other less pressure-filled and demanding specialties.

The young patient was treated less vigorously than is usual for the ICU. For example, he was not placed on a ventilator to help him breathe, although this is often done in the ICU with patients in whom the indications are much more dubious. Thus the doctors substantiated the self-fulfilling prophecy that the patient would not benefit from the ICU. In fact, his doctor was called and told that his patient was dying; if he did not arrange for the patient to be transferred back to his care, they would see to it that the patient was delivered bodily to him.

This highly unusual behavior greatly disturbed the orthopedic surgeon. He went to the ICU to see his patient. He found him fatigued from the effort to breathe and doing badly; he clearly needed a ventilator to support life. When the request for the use of a ventilator was denied on the grounds that the 19-year-old patient was doomed and should be left to die in peace, his doctor enlisted the help of a senior physician on the hospital staff. When this physician saw the patient he insisted that he be placed on a ventilator. He reasoned as follows:

· The patient was only 19 years old and it was necessary to give him every chance to survive.
· The ICU doctors had no real experience with patients suffering from muscular dystrophy and were applying their observations of patients with chronic lung disease to a patient with chronic muscle disease. No one, including the ICU doctors, really knew how patients with muscular dystrophy might respond to treatment.
· Lack of oxygen makes muscles work less effectively. Perhaps improving the level of oxygen in the blood by using a ventilator would result in improved respiratory muscle function.
· The breathing muscles of the patient were obviously fatigued and use of a ventilator might rest them.

The disagreement over placing the patient on a ventilator was not resolved by sweet reason. The senior physician had his way because he shouted louder and commanded more authority. The patient was placed on a ventilator and made a rapid and remarkable recovery. His story has a happy ending worth sharing. The young man went on to college and graduated four years later, at age 23.

This episode illustrates how difficult it can be to decide that a patient is terminally ill. If any doubt exists, the decision should be in favor of treatment, but when a clear diagnosis of terminal illness can be made, the patient should not be admitted to the ICU. Such a decision, however, has serious psychological and ethical implications for both the physicians and the family. As a result, many patients are admitted to ICUs who, because they are dying of nontreatable causes, cannot possibly benefit from care in the ICU.

What should the admission policy be for patients who are "no code"—those for whom no attempt at cardiopulmonary resuscitation will be made if the heart ceases beating, because they are considered terminally ill? Some argue that the a priori decision to let the patient die under one circumstance (cardiac arrest) indicates that the patient is not salvageable and that a decision to exclude him from the ICU should automatically follow. Others contend that the two decisions may not be closely linked—that each decision should be made separately. There is no clear-cut answer.

You may well ask, Is there no way patients can die a comfortable and dignified death in the ICU, if this appears to be in their best interest? The answer is that the atmosphere does not easily lend itself to compassionate and careful analysis. Policy dictates that all patients in the ICU receive very intense treatment. ICUs are dedicated to aggressive, invasive, and extensive intervention. The ICU is committed not only to the care of the critically ill, *but to taking care of them intensively,* whether or not this is in their best interests. It can be concluded that the ICU is not a good place to die gracefully.

Iatrogenics in the ICU

Some patients develop complications or die *as a result* of having been admitted to an ICU. The size of this group is not known for individual units, but that it is substantial can be inferred from what data are available. One study indicates that, in the critically ill, major complications of treatment—life-threatening complications—develop in one-fifth to one-third of all patients.

Several factors contribute to the extraordinarily high rate of iatrogenic episodes in ICUs. An attempt to salvage critically ill patients may require aggressive treatment—"desperate diseases require desperate measures." A wide variety of interventions may be tried, each with its inherent risks. Innovations in management, some of dubious value, are often too hastily used in patients, a practice that contributes to a high rate of complications.

For example, a test commonly used in the ICU measures blood pressure in the lungs by the use of a Swan-Ganz catheter. In a few selected patients the test is of value, but in most patients its value is dubious. It is nevertheless enthusiastically used in the ICU.

A recently published study established that more accurate information of certain kinds can be obtained by the use of the Swan-Ganz catheter than by the performance of a history and a physical examination. But the question to be addressed is, Does the use of the catheter lead to a better outcome for patients? The authors admitted that their study did not address this important issue. Their results are similar to the discovery that witchcraft is a better treatment for cancer than are the bladders of toads.

If there were no risks in using the Swan-Ganz catheter, this study, which, like many studies, asked the wrong questions, might not be important. A small but significant number of complications, however, do result from the use of the Swan-Ganz catheter, including death. Given these definite risks, to publish such a study might be considered harmful; it is often cited and has probably increased the inappropriate use of the technique.

Responses to ICU Treatment

There is a subgroup of patients in whom iatrogenic episodes represent a major risk; these are the patients who are not so critically ill but who are managed in the ICU as if they are. Nondesperate diseases should be treated with nondesperate measures, but this principle is apt to be overlooked in the ICU.

For example, patients with cardiac pulmonary edema—too much water in the lung because of heart disease—can be managed adequately in an ordinary medical ward, but they are increasingly treated in the ICU. Often they are placed on breathing machines much more frequently than would seem necessary and are thereby subjected to high risks of complications. The same is true of patients with bronchial asthma and pneumonia.

Some patients are now actually admitted to ICUs merely because the equipment for a particular measurement is available only there. To some extent, this need is being met by creating ICUs based on gradations of severity of illness. So-called "intermediate" ICUs are for patients less critically ill than those who are admitted to regular ICUs. Perhaps we will soon have "moderate" intensive care units, similar to ordinary medical wards. And ultimately, who knows, we may have "minimal" intensive care units, in which the patient is kept at home.

There is another group of patients who would have died or developed complications independently of the ICU. Iatrogenic complications are found in all areas of a hospital.

There is a group of patients who would recover in or out of an ICU but are subjected to the increased risk of ICU treatment without distinct benefits.

Finally, there is a group of patients who do better specifically because they are treated in the ICU. The basic purpose of the ICU is, of course, to raise the number in this group as much as possible.

The Benefits of ICU Management

How effective are the individual diagnostic and therapeutic measures performed in an ICU? No one knows. Increased monitoring of patients for a wide variety of different body functions has become the rule in ICU management, but the value of this extensive monitoring in terms of improved patient outcome is not known. It is pursued in the hope that its benefits outweigh its risks.

Of the numerous forms of treatment used in patients in the ICU, very few can be scientifically justified and almost none have been shown to improve patient outcome.

Here is a true-to-life (or death) scenario, commonly acted out in an ICU: The senior physician on the morning rounds reviews a given treatment; it is his judgment that the treatment is helpful. The senior physician in charge of the afternoon shift judges that the same treatment is harmful. But when the senior physician on evening duty reviews the same treatment, he suggests that the two other senior doctors are wrong and recommends a completely different approach. This occurs without anyone being aware that one expert is saying "white," another is saying "black," and a third is saying "gray."

It is well known that medical advice with regard to the same medical problem often differs dramatically from expert to expert. These differences of opinion, recorded and played back to the patient whose fate is being decided, would produce the most profound anxieties. But most doctors take this amazing phenomenon in stride without drawing the obvious conclusion: Medical practice is pragmatic and often has no solid foundation. For many problems, there is no single answer; for many, there is no satisfactory answer.

And what do intensivists themselves think about the value of ICUs? A recent consensus conference to consider this question arrived at a curious conclusion: Although the value of ICUs and the various forms of treatment could not be supported by hard facts, the units were of value. The endorsement was presumably based on faith, which, as we have seen, can move doctors as well as mountains.

The Coronary Care Unit (CCU)

Like the ICU, the CCU is a specially designated, geographically distinct area of the hospital. It was established to provide specialized care for patients with heart attacks, and a team of specially trained physicians and nurses looks after these patients. The CCU contains specialized equipment for monitoring various heart functions as well as specialized equipment used to treat various malfunctions.

These units were first established in the 1960s in an attempt to decrease mortality from heart attacks. The sickest patients often do not survive to reach the unit. Perhaps 50 percent of all deaths occur within the first hour after a heart attack and 65 percent within the first 12 hours. The medical system has enlarged its ability to help early victims of heart attacks: The training of paramedical personnel—firemen, policemen, specially trained "medics," and lay people—in cardiopulmonary resuscitation (CPR) has made for decreases in early death rates. Specially trained "medics" (non-doctors trained in emergency treatment) are a valuable addition to the medical system. The benefits of having available such a group exceed the risks involved.

The original objective was to deal with important causes of death following heart attacks—cardiac arrest, in which the heart stops beating, and cardiac bradytachyarrhythmias, in which the heart beats too slowly, too rapidly, or too irregularly to pump blood adequately. Use of the CCU was then extended to the detection and treatment of other potentially lethal effects of heart attack. One of these is cardiogenic shock —decreased blood pressure because of damage to the heart muscle; and another is cardiogenic pulmonary edema—excess water in the lungs due to the inability of the heart to pump adequate amounts of blood.

Finally, its use was extended to patients who may or may not have had a heart attack. As with all diseases, the manifestations may not be specific. Signs resembling those of a heart attack characterize a number of other quite different diseases. Some of these are benign and usually heal without major morbidity or mortality. For example, the pericardium may be infected by a virus and give rise to chest pain difficult to distinguish from that experienced in a heart attack.

CCUs developed and proliferated to an amazing degree, and most hospitals have their own CCU. You will not be surprised to learn that this occurred without any acceptable preliminary studies to indicate that the units provided more benefits than risks.

What are some of the limitations of the CCU? The overtreatment of patients tends to be the rule in such units. For example, a heart attack provokes a disturbance of heart rhythm known as ventricular premature beats—extra heartbeats arising from the heart muscle. In many or most patients this disturbance is transient and corrects itself. But in a few patients it may herald the development of more extensive rhythm disturbances, and these can lead to death. In the CCU, the ventricular premature beats are usually detected by an electronic monitor and treated with various drugs which in themselves can produce severe complications. Recent attempts have been made to identify the precise types of premature beats that require treatment with drugs. A careful clinical trial will ultimately be required to validate these attempts.

Some studies have suggested that CCUs salvage more patients than they harm, and others suggest the reverse. In England, one study divided patients into three groups: One-third were treated in a CCU, one-third in an ordinary ward of the hospital, and one-third at home. The death rate was lowest among those treated at home! The difference in death rates did not appear to reflect any differences in degrees of illness among the groups—or to suggest that the sickest patients went to the hospital and the least sick stayed at home.

Similar results were reported in another study from England and in one from Canada. Yet another study compared the outcome of patients admitted to a CCU with those admitted to an ordinary ward and could detect no differences in outcome.

Why might patients in a CCU do less well than those treated at home or in an ordinary ward? Obviously because they are less likely to be overdiagnosed and overtreated on an ordinary ward than they would be in a CCU. It has also been suggested that the isolation of a CCU and the anxiety it provokes actually cause disturbances of heart rhythm and other problems, and thus tend to increase morbidity and mortality. The issue is by no means settled and may never be adequately studied.

One favorable review of the value of CCUs concludes that it is the *conviction* of physicians, rather than a conclusion drawn from firm statistical evidence, that the CCU prevents deaths from heart attacks, and this conviction has led to the wide use of CCUs.

The Unavoidable Question

As a potential patient, how will you make a choice if and when it becomes necessary? Will you accept or reject the care of an ICU or CCU? If you become terminally ill you will have to decide how you prefer to die. These words do not even suggest the agony involved in such a difficult decision. But if you do not deal with it yourself, the decision will by default be made by physicians who cannot share your feelings and are therefore less competent to decide.

If you are a close relative or friend of someone who must face this decision, you will have to do your best to carry out the patient's wishes. If the patient has not made or cannot make these wishes explicitly known to you, you will have to rely on your insight. The question to ask yourself is, What would the patient have wanted? The question the doctor should ask you is, What would the patient have wanted? If you decide that a heroic, but probably useless, stay in the ICU does not meet the wishes of your friend or relative, you should not feel guilty about keeping him out of the ICU. We all feel guilty when someone close to us dies; that is probably inevitable, but it need not deter us from making the decision we believe is right.

If it is proposed that you be admitted to an ICU, you should, when possible, make it your business to learn why. Try to be certain that the proposal is based on precise indications, that it is not made simply because the ICU is the conventional site to treat your illness.

If you are suspected of having a heart attack, try to spend as little time as possible in a CCU. This is probably good advice even if you are a definite heart attack victim. Keep track of the studies being performed on you, so that you are informed about your specific situation. Remember that the history of treatment of heart attacks in this country provides little support for the view that the doctor always knows best. Treatment of heart attacks has gradually changed from several months, to six weeks in bed in a hospital, to six weeks in a bed and chair, to relatively early ambulation and early discharge. There is reason to maintain some degree of reservation about inflexible advice.

If, on the other hand, you have any of the complications associated with heart attacks, then the hospital is the best place for you. If coronary surgery is proposed as part of your treatment, try to discover why this is recommended for you. If a new form of nonoperative treatment is proposed—thrombolytic therapy, in which drugs are used to attempt to dissolve blood clots in the coronary vessels—recognize that such studies are still experimental. Decide whether you want to participate in the experiment.

Remember that the general effectiveness of ICUs and CCUs has not been established; only in certain specialized groups of patients has a favorable balance between risk and benefit been documented. The atmosphere and pace of ICUs create medical complications for greater numbers of patients than do other sites in the hospital. The less critically ill patient is at special risk. In fact, some studies indicate that patients with uncomplicated heart attacks do better when treated at home than in the CCU.

To summarize, the high-risk groups needlessly in the ICU are the dying, who suffer a loss of dignity and excess discomfort as a result of treatment, and the not-so-critically ill, who are exposed to the extra risks of ICU care with little possibility of benefit.

The Essence of Critical Care

The ICU and CCU have become self-perpetuating—in part because patients believe in them, in part because doctors are attracted by the drama, the intellectual excitement, and the medical challenge they offer. The experience that proves too intensive for the patient may be intensely interesting to the doctor. This anecdote can be taken as typical of a young doctor's reaction to the ICU.

"That's a great case," says one medical resident to another in the ICU. He is describing a patient whose skin is covered with a rash, whose legs are horribly ulcerated, who is yellowed by jaundice because her liver has failed, whose lungs are filled with fluid, whose heart is failing, and who is unconscious because of abnormal brain function. She is "a great case" because she represents an intellectual and medical challenge. As he leaves the ICU, the young doctor changes mental gears; his manner reflects dignified sadness as he reports to the patient's children that she probably will not survive. This young doctor is not a hypocrite. He is genuine in his response to the medical challenge and genuine in his compassion.

11

The Terminally Ill and the Aged

Death is an inevitable consequence of life. We must all face the prospect of becoming terminally ill at some point in our lives. In reality, this prospect confronts us from the very inception of life, as we all begin to die at that moment. We go through a stage in which we are terminally well until a rapid or slow transition takes place and we become terminally ill.

These abstract musings do have practical implications. One is that a life spent worrying about death or being obsessed with the possibility of disease cannot be particularly happy or productive and is not to be recommended. The other is that when life-threatening illness occurs may be time enough to consider how to deal with the specifics of mortality.

This is not to say that one should ignore matters such as life insurance or providing for one's family. But the specific details of one's final illness should not be an obsessive concern: When it occurs each of us will be faced with certain decisions and so will our doctors.

For the doctor there are especially vexing problems and grave responsibilities associated with the care of the terminally ill. As we have seen, defining a terminal state may be difficult. The young patient with muscular dystrophy discussed in Chapter 10 was prematurely diagnosed as terminally ill. Appropriately treated, he went from terminally ill to terminally well.

On the other hand, patients judged terminally ill may recover when treatment is withdrawn. Four patients in a surgical ICU were considered terminally ill. To allow them greater comfort in the remaining limited period of life, their doctors decided to withdraw all treatment except for intravenous fluid. No more drugs were given, no special treatments were permitted, no more tests were run. Two of the four patients rallied; their temperature became normal, they began to eat, regained some muscle strength, and were discharged home to lead some kind of productive life. This episode illustrates two important issues, both of which deserve emphasis: The potential error in defining a patient as terminal and the possibility that treatment itself may accelerate terminal illness.

The terminally ill patient who defies expectations and survives longer than the time predicted may develop a second, unrelated illness, which, if treated, may temporarily improve life. For example, a given patient with a very aggressive metastatic cancer of the breast will almost certainly die within months. She develops severe bleeding from her gastrointestinal tract. Should she undergo surgery to treat the bleeding? Should she be given massive blood transfusions? Should she be treated only enough to keep her comfortable while she is "permitted" to bleed to death? These are extraordinarily difficult questions for which there can be no simple or universal answers.

Evolving Definitions of Death

If defining terminal illness is difficult, defining death is in some instances equally or more difficult. In the United States, death is usually defined as brain death, but different parts of the brain die at different rates. For example, the brain stem—the lower part of the brain that regulates breathing and the action of the heart—tends to die more slowly than those higher parts of the brain responsible for intellect and emotion and for the generation of the brain waves recorded by electro-encephalography (EEG). Because of this difference in rate, a patient may have upper brain death while the lower brain continues to function.

The case of Karen Anne Quinlan, who, for reasons not fully known, became unconscious, has been widely publicized. In an ICU, her life was supported by a ventilator, fluids, and other measures. She neither moved nor responded to stimuli; her brain waves were virtually flat. A long legal battle was waged over whether to "pull the plug." If to withdraw the support system was legally proper, who would take responsibility for the decision? After much deliberation the courts decided that it was proper to stop ventilatory support. This was done, and the patient continued to breathe on her own— her upper brain had died but her lower brain continued to function and to sustain her breathing.

The primary role in determining treatment of the terminally ill often falls to the doctor. The doctor is on the scene as life begins to ebb. As the most authoritative figure present, he must make the judgment that the patient is or is not terminally ill. Until recently, a simple principle was exercised: Aggressive medical treatment should be continued up to the moment of death at any cost. Until methods for keeping the near-dead alive for long periods became available, the questions that now arise from invoking that principle were largely academic. That prolongation of life was always in the best interest of the patient was taken for granted.

A dramatic change has occurred: Society and the medical system have concluded that the dying need not be kept alive indefinitely. But because no coherent set of rules has evolved as a guide to the decisions that now become necessary, the doctor's domain has been extended beyond the medical. The doctor now becomes the arbiter, although the courts have maintained that under some circumstances the final decision is within their jurisdiction.

How competent are doctors to decide whether to continue or to withdraw treatment in the terminally ill? Not very. No acceptable theoretical basis exists for these decisions. The issues involved are not amenable to medical or technological solutions or to scientific analysis; any theory advanced is merely the opinion of one expert or another. No formulas have evolved; no scientific studies have provided a solution.

In practice, however, doctors often act as though there were rules. Applied mechanically, these supposed rules lead to some grotesque decisions. A patient suffered brain damage when his breathing stopped following surgery. A group of doctors agreed that irreversible brain damage had occurred. Informed that withdrawal of treatment was warranted on the basis of expert opinion, the family consented. All treatment, including nutrients, was stopped, and the patient died.

This case was reviewed by a group of experts that included some nationally known figures. They could not conclude with any certainty that the patient had suffered irreversible brain damage. They were certain, however, that such damage had not been documented. Had life been maintained for another few weeks until the potential for reversibility could be determined, at the very least the family could have been spared the pain and guilt of a possibly incorrect and certainly premature decision.

Were the doctors malicious or evil? Not at all. They thought they were acting in the best interests of the patient and his family. They had learned that irreversible brain death was an indication for stopping treatment. They had not learned how easy it may be to make an error in judgment. It is difficult to support the view that, in these situations, "the doctor knows best."

The Patient's Right to Decide

The ultimate judgment is not fundamentally a technical or medical matter, and the decision to continue or abandon treatment is not within the doctor's province. When the decision is left to the doctor, the risk is that the patient's deepest desires will be violated. The final answer can be found only in the human heart and can be determined only on an individual basis. There is no body of information from which doctors can be taught to make judgments that will predictably serve the best interests of each terminally ill patient. The doctor should serve as a medical advisor, as a consultant, and perhaps as a friend. For the decision to be made by anyone but the patient or close family at the time of death is a violation of the most fundamental rights of patients.

That this principle can work is well illustrated by the thoughtful approach to patients with severe burns devised by one hospital in the United States. The burn treatment unit in this hospital has accumulated extensive data on the relationship between the amount of body surface burned and the likelihood of survival. Gathered under conditions characterized by highly aggressive and intensive care of burn victims, these data show that when burns involve more than a given portion of the body surface, recovery is unlikely. With this information, it is possible to estimate the probability of survival for patients given all-out treatment. This does not mean that every patient whose burned area exceeds a given value will die. Nor does it mean that every patient with a smaller burn area will survive. The data provide the best *guess* as to the outcome.

Upon admission to the hospital, a patient whose burns exceed in body surface that amount usually associated with survival is offered the choice of conventional intensive treatment with its attendant pain, discomfort, loss of dignity, and other problems, or the alternative choice of minimal supportive therapy with patient comfort as the major goal.

The patient is allowed adequate time to reach a decision, to consult anyone who can help—relatives, friends, religious advisors. During the relatively pain-free interval following a burn—the nerve endings for pain in the afflicted area are destroyed by the burn—the patient can more easily make a rational decision. That decision, however, is not irrevocable; when patients change their minds, and they often do, their management is changed accordingly.

This approach was developed to fit the circumstances associated with burns and may not be practical extended to other situations, but it is sensitive and sensible. It recognizes the primary right of the patient to decide his own fate. It relegates the doctor to the role of medical advisor and provider of care. It offers realistic alternatives to patients who are dying at a time when they are still able to make their own decision. It is done with great honesty and the principle of patient autonomy is beautifully preserved.

Care of the Aged

There are two good reasons why the need for medical care increases with age: One, aging is accompanied by a series of changes, part of an inexorable process, that diminish physical and mental capacity. Although these occur at different rates in different people, with the passage of time they take place in everyone. Two, the old are especially susceptible to a number of diseases, among them heart diseases, diseases of blood vessels, and various forms of cancer. Their need for medical care is therefore more urgent than that of younger people.

The medical system is not especially designed to meet the medical problems of the aged. The emergence of geriatrics as a medical specialty is an important step forward, in that we now have doctors especially sensitive to the needs of the aging. But these specialists are dependent upon the same experts and are subject to the limitations of the same medical system that serves the general population.

Old people are subject to the same risks as other patients, but for them these risks assume special forms. Overdiagnosis and overtreatment are quite common in the old, just as they are in other age groups, but, paradoxically, undertreatment may be practiced because the patient is considered too old to be given acceptable care. The following case is an example.

An 84-year-old man is a functional and relatively happy person. He works at home as a stockbroker, loves watching sports on television, and is involved in life. He develops some muscle pain in the rib cage as a result of strenuous physical activity. The pain is minor but annoying. He consults a physician and is treated with a drug known to be associated with the development of stomach ulcers.

Early one morning he awakens with excruciating abdominal pain unlike the original pain. He calls his doctor, who downplays the importance of the new pain and suggests that the patient take codeine for his pain. The patient persists in calling and finally the doctor agrees to an office visit. The patient is examined; he is obviously in great distress and quite ill. His doctor has no explanation for the pain. The patient wants to be admitted to a hospital. His doctor informs him, "If you insist I'll admit you, but are you certain that you want to be hospitalized?" The patient persists. On admission to the hospital, he is found to have a perforated stomach. The rupture occurred through a stomach ulcer almost certainly caused by the medication prescribed by the doctor for the original episode of rib cage pain.

The stomach is repaired in surgery and, despite a somewhat stormy hospital course, he recovers and returns home to resume a satisfactory life. Had the patient not insisted on being hospitalized, he would have died. The patient understands the issues all too well. He is bitterly resentful that his doctor almost sentenced him to death by resisting his decision to be hospitalized.

Several errors were committed. One was to underestimate the degree of illness on the basis of telephone conversations —an error that could be made by any doctor; it had little to do with the patient's age. Then the doctor badly misjudged the patient's will to survive. He also misjudged the vitality of his patient, reasoning that 84-year-olds are so close to death that invasive procedures should not be considered. That may be true of many 84-year-olds but certainly not of all. Every 84-year-old is unique.

That necessary medical care may be withheld merely on the basis of age is a special risk that the old face. Errors in the opposite direction, however, occur much more frequently. Overdiagnosis and overtreatment probably prevail more commonly among the old than among other patients, undoubtedly because the old are more exposed to doctors than are other age groups. We have already seen some instances of this: the 74-year-old woman subjected to an open-lung biopsy for lung disease (Chapter 4) is one. The 83-year-old woman with cancer of the breast who was subjected to endoscopy because of upper gastrointestinal bleeding (Chapter 3) is another.

A 75-year-old woman developed heartburn and mild persistent stomach pain after the death of her husband. Antacids and tranquilizers relieved her symptoms, but she underwent an x-ray of her esophagus, stomach, and small bowel, and an x-ray and ultrasound examination of her gall-bladder, to determine whether she had a peptic ulcer or gallbladder disease. Another test measured the function of her liver, and a multitude of routine tests (blood count, urinalysis, electrocardiogram, chest x-ray, blood chemistry measurements) were done for reasons that are not clear. Most of the testing took place after her symptoms had largely cleared up. The same workup might be considered too extreme for a 25-year-old patient; it was certainly too extreme for a 75-year-old.

A 78-year-old woman with mild heart disease and a degree of senility was maintained on some 20 different drugs—heart drugs, pain killers, tranquilizers, anticoagulants, etc. Some served to protect against the effects of others. Because of her senility she was unable to keep the drugs straight. As a result she chronically overdosed and underdosed herself. She was hospitalized and the number of medicines reduced from twenty to five, at which point her physical state markedly improved. Even young patients get into trouble through the excessive use of medicine, but these difficulties tend to be more extreme in the old.

A medical journal editorializes, "The evidence stands overwhelmingly against the routine annual physical except possibly for older men." Why the exception for older men? Presumably because the prevalence of certain diseases is higher in this group. But the harmful impact of the annual physicals themselves might well fall most heavily on the older age group. One of the risks of these examinations is that they report false positives. There is no evidence that the incidence of false positives is lower in the old, and they have less time remaining to spend in medical dead ends or potentially harmful medical encounters.

Chronological Versus Physiological Age

Doctors employ an interesting concept in deciding on invasive forms of treatment for the aged—a distinction between chronological age and physiological age. Chronological age is obviously fixed at the actual age of the patient. Physiological age, however, is the doctor's estimate of how physically vigorous the patient may be. An extensive surgical procedure was being considered in an 87-year-old patient. In justifying the operation, the surgeon stated that the patient was physiologically much younger than his actual 87 years. An internist who doubted the need for surgery stated that the patient was older than his actual 87 years. Such evaluations are largely subjective; the physiological age of the patient is frequently in the eye of the observer.

Special Risks for the Aged

The aged patient faces special risks.

* Doctors may not realize that in planning care for the aged they should anticipate fewer total years of survival than in younger patients. Even a healthy 70-year-old patient has statistically few years to live, say an average of five more years. A 35-year-old patient has perhaps 40 years remaining. Diagnostic and therapeu-

tic measures in the aged should be geared to this reality. Approaches appropriate to the older patient may be quite different from the approaches to a younger patient with the same problem.

- The time spent in the hospital or in convalescence deprives the aged of a greater percentage of their remaining life than it does the young. For a 30-year-old patient, one uncomfortable, unproductive month represents a potential loss of 1/540th of remaining life; the same period of time would represent 1/60th of remaining life for a 70-year-old. The impact of management should therefore be more carefully estimated for the old.
- Old people tolerate changes in the condition of life less well than the young. The transition from home life to hospital life tends to be more disruptive in the old.
- Old people tend to have more physical complications from treatment than young people. For example, complication rates following surgery in the old are much higher than they are in younger patients. For any given medical problem the old should be treated more conservatively than the young.

When age or illness forces you, as a patient or as a close relative or friend of a patient, to deal with the difficult and complex problems of terminal illness or the illnesses of old age, how will you reach the necessary decisions? It is my strong opinion that the ultimate decision *belongs to the patient.* I do not believe that the courts have a primary role to play. Issues with societal overtones so complex that they can only be decided legally should occur rarely. Only the patient can evaluate the illness and treatment in terms of his deepest feelings.

If the patient is not in a position to make the decision, then this right belongs to the patient's family, who should base their decision on their interpretation of the patient's wishes; if the family is not available, then to a surrogate who would presumably have been acceptable to the patient. For assistance with the medical issues involved, family and friends are well advised to turn to an ombudsdoctor. If none of these persons is available, then the doctor may be forced to make the decision —with humility and with the understanding that his decision may be incorrect and may violate the deepest feelings of the patient.

12

Making Patients out of Normal Human Beings

"An ounce of prevention is worth a pound of cure." That it is wise to identify and intervene in health problems as soon as possible seems obvious, and this bit of folk wisdom is strongly ingrained in medicine. In practice, however, it conflicts with the sage advice of Benjamin Franklin that "nothing is more fatal to health than overcare of it."

The first aphorism has provided the conceptual basis for much of modern medical care and is perhaps best exemplified in the health survey, periodic checkup, and screening test. A health survey can vary from an exhaustive examination, such as multiphasic screening, to a single test for a single disease. Screening means that large numbers of apparently normal people are tested for a specific abnormality. An annual checkup is a collection of screening tests. A growing number of doctors are challenging the value of health surveys in the normal (healthy) person on two grounds: Their inherent risks and the lack of evidence to prove their benefits.

The Risks and Benefits of Health Care Surveys

Having read this far, you can name some of the potential risks of health care surveys. For every participant, they create a distraction from the main issues of life; in the healthy, these should not include illness. The harm to the true negatives, those pronounced free of disease, is that they will undergo needless additional studies. The greater harm, of course, is to the false negatives—those who are spuriously reassured that they do not have an illness which in fact they do have.

The true positives—those whose illness is uncovered—benefit only if the illness can be effectively treated, and if treating the disease at an early stage improves the outcome. The false positives—those who are told they are ill when in fact they are not—suffer the greatest harm. They are subjected to all of the risks that true-positive patients must face. Inevitably, they suffer some degree of emotional trauma; the more serious the supposed disease, the more severe the trauma. Because it is difficult to measure psychological harm, this consequence is underemphasized or ignored. The original test is generally followed by a series of additional tests, each with its own hazards, frequently with morbidity and mortality. Unnecessary expense is probably the least important of the hazards, but ultimately you may pay to have yourself killed by being managed for a disease you do not have.

Some Benefits of Surveys

On the other hand, a serious disease may be revealed by the test at an early and treatable stage. The possible early detection of disease is not the only benefit that health surveys offer normal people. A screening survey may serve as an introduction to valuable medical care, including immunization by vaccines. A presumed benefit of screening is that it provides a baseline value at a time when the subject is healthy. A comparison with the result of the same test when the patient is ill can be of substantial value. For example, interpretation of an x-ray is more accurate if it can be compared to an earlier x-ray. An earlier electrocardiogram may help the doctor in interpreting an electrocardiogram obtained when a patient is ill. This reasoning, however, could lead to the performance of every conceivable test on every subject and ignores the risks of testing. Finally, the doctor, hospital, or clinic conducting the survey will keep medical records for you so that they can theoretically be available when you become ill.

The Special Risks for the Healthy

Before you submit to any screening test when you are not obviously ill, you need to know the probability of a helpful versus a harmful outcome. How can the balance between the risks and benefits be determined?

You have already learned that such an analysis can be made *only* by means of a careful and well-designed prospective clinical trial in which the fate of those being tested is compared with that of a group who do not undergo the test. For most tests used in surveys of normal subjects no such trials have been made, and millions of subjects are undergoing tests that may have an unfavorable risk-benefit ratio. To establish this ratio is even more critical in testing normals than in testing patients. The patient is like someone who has been hit by an automobile while crossing the street. He *has* to be treated and must accept the potential risks along with the potential benefits of treatment. The normal subject has been *pushed* in front of the car. The harm to him has been a consequence of external intervention.

How Surveys Evolve

The doctors and health professionals who advocate and perform health surveys are attempting to improve the health of the community. The organizations who endorse and sponsor surveys are among the most public-spirited groups in society. Surveys are usually directed by experts in the specific areas of disease encompassed by the survey. How is it possible that they would lend their support to projects whose risk factors are unknown? The answer is that if a survey has been traditionally used, they assume that it is valid and therefore do not subject it to adequate review; nor do they question the data on which it is based. Data that conflict with the preconceived notion that the survey is effective are usually ignored, and the few experts who may call attention to deficiencies are usually ignored as well.

Because the scientific basis for a survey is often so tenuous, major shifts in policy are frequent. Fluoroscopy of the chest, annual chest x-rays, and pulmonary-function testing have been used on millions of normals and then abandoned. Examination of sputum to detect cancer of the lung in normal subjects has come and gone. The recommended annual cervical Pap smear has given way to the periodic Pap smear. Recommendations for mammography have gone through a series of changes. How many patients had an open-lung biopsy because of a false-positive finding of cancer in the sputum—a now discarded form of survey? No one knows. How many of them suffered postoperative complications? No one knows. How many of them died? No one knows. The victims of the now discarded approach do not receive an apology for having been mishandled.

Failure to obtain data is usually rationalized. "Too many patients will die of this disease if we delay the survey until we can perform adequate clinical trials. It would be unethical to delay the survey." Is it more ethical to have false positives die needlessly? Other arguments against clinical trials are: Most doctors will not support the performance of clinical trials; volunteers will not participate; the design of clinical trials is too difficult; clinical trials are too costly. But in the absence of the information that acceptable clinical trials would generate, there can be no adequate risk-benefit assessment; prospective subjects cannot make an informed choice about participating; and doctors cannot give accurate advice as to whether patients should participate.

Criteria for Effective Surveys

The World Health Organization, recognizing the need to establish risk-benefit ratios for health surveys, has suggested a series of criteria for an effective survey of an individual disease in normal populations.

1. The condition should be an important health problem for masses of people. [The benefits of diagnosing trivial diseases would not justify expending the resources or taking risks.]

2. There should be an accepted treatment for patients with a recognized disease. [This criterion is crucial. The only justifiable reason for screening healthy patients is to keep them healthy. Many surveys screen for diseases that are untreatable.]

3. Facilities for diagnosis and treatment should be available. [Without these, the results of the test cannot be translated into proper treatment.]

4. There should be a recognizable latent, or early symptomatic, stage of the disease. [The point of the survey is to pick up disease at an early stage in the hope of improving the outlook by early treatment.]

5. There should be a suitable test or examination. [Many tests are not sufficiently sensitive, or specific, or accurate.]

6. The test should be acceptable to the population. [If not, it would be impractical to attempt to conduct the survey.]

7. The natural history of the condition, including development from latent to overt disease, should be adequately understood. [If not, intervention by doctors might be meddlesome.]

8. There should be an agreed-upon policy as to whom to treat as patients. [If not, the test might identify

large numbers of subjects who would not be eligible for treatment.]

9. The cost of the survey, including diagnosis and treatment, should be economically balanced in relation to the cost of medical care as a whole.

10. The finding of cases should be an ongoing process and not a once-and-for-all project. [If the survey is valuable, it should provide health benefits over a long period of time.]

The World Health Organization concluded that *none* of the screening tests in common use during the 1960s met all of these requirements! There have been no significant advances since that time. We can only conclude that innumerable normal subjects have been screened, and are being screened, by approaches that are at best inadequately evaluated and at worst harmful.

But even the criteria fixed by the World Health Organization are insufficient. They deal only with the direct application of the test. They assume the scientific and technical validity of the given test and the usefulness of its data as applied to suitable subjects.

A number of other requirements should be met before widespread application of any test in normals.

1. The results of the test should show acceptable reproducibility. This means that if the same measurement is repeated several times without changing any of the conditions of the test, the results of the measurement will all be close to each other.

2. For tests that generate observer interpretations rather than numbers (x-rays, scans, evaluation of the nature of cells, etc.), the variation of interpretation among a number of expert observers should be small. At present, for some or most tests of this type individual interpretations vary widely, so that the results are largely subjective and unreliable.

3. The test should be subjected to a pilot trial on a small segment of a population whose composition is similar to that of the population ultimately to be screened. A lack of similarity may result in major interpretive errors, so that if a large population is studied, many subjects may be injured before the potential harm is detected. In this pilot trial, the sensitivity of the test (a measure of which is the percent of false negatives), the specificity of the test (a measure of which is the percent of false positives), and the accuracy of the test should be determined. All of these values are essential to an accurate analysis of the risks versus benefits of a given screening procedure. (See glossary for technical definitions.)

4. After the procedure is introduced into general use, the subjects in the pilot trial should be observed for a period of time sufficient to reveal whether the test in question is likely to benefit the general population and sufficient to allow any unexpected long-term hazards to emerge.

5. The impact of the test on the well-being of false positives should be followed over a long period of time. The false positives are the hidden victims of surveys of apparently normal populations. This cannot be overemphasized.

These five requirements are seldom, if ever, met. We really know little about the usefulness of even well-established screening tests and procedures. Instead, we have the "recommendations" of experts, which amount to opinions or guesses.

Careful evaluation of tests in surveys admittedly poses a familiar dilemma. If a test can be evaluated only over a long period of time, its benefits may be denied to a large number of people. On the other hand, if careful evaluation is not performed, the public is subject to needless or harmful procedures.

As a potential candidate for a wide variety of testing procedures, you should know that, for most of them, adequate *scientific* justification has not been established. Should you decide to participate in such surveys, you will at least know that your participation is not an unmixed blessing.

Let us now examine some specific forms of screening in normal populations.

The Periodic or Annual Health Checkup

For decades the periodic health examination has been seen as a useful form of health care in the United States. It now turns out that there is no acceptable data base establishing its usefulness as a general approach. This does not rule out the possibility that, were studies done, the benefits might be found to outweigh the risks, but it does indicate that its advocates should validate its effectiveness before it is used, as there is a strong possibility that it can result in harm to normal subjects.

A Reassessment

Available evidence suggests that general health examinations are not useful. Over a period of 12 years, ending in 1982, the Kaiser-Permanente Prepaid Health Plan conducted a controlled, randomized clinical trial of general health evaluation. Five thousand adults were regularly screened and 5,000, the controls, were not. In terms of outcome as to major disabilities, improvement in the rates of chronic diseases, or mortality, the data showed insignificant differences between the group undergoing periodic examinations and the control group.* Similar findings have been reported from Utah; Van-

---

*A separate analysis found some benefits for the routine use of sigmoidoscopy in decreasing the death rate from cancer of the colon or rectum. These data are, in my opinion, inadequate to support the conclusion that sigmoidoscopy reduced the death rate from cancer. The data did not consider the harm to subjects who were false positives.

couver, Canada; Edinburgh, Scotland; and Adelaide, Australia. The Australian study found that screening did not favorably affect mortality, length of hospital stay, disability and distress suffered by patients, or speed in initiating treatment for detected abnormalities.

These studies have uniformly failed to demonstrate the benefit of periodic examinations. Summations such as "The evidence stands overwhelmingly against the routine annual physical examination, except possibly for older men," summarize the views of most thoughtful observers concerning periodic health screening.

Supporting evidence comes from the conclusions of A Task Force in the Periodic Health Examination set up by the Canadian government. This group did not attempt specifically to analyze the effect of various studies on patient health. Nor did they concern themselves with risks versus benefits. Rather, they focused on the accuracy of detection and the incidence of the various diseases targeted by the tests. They concluded that few of the routine examination procedures made sense in terms of early detection or prevention of disease.

The Canadian group recommended that a number of standard tests be eliminated from periodic routine examinations: urinalyses, electrocardiograms, measurements of blood chemical constituents, and routine x-ray examinations such as the chest x-ray. Even the blood count was eliminated except in certain high-risk groups. They found little or no value in the taking of a medical history in normal subjects. They did, however, recommend mammograms for women aged 50 to 60.

New Technology, New Tests, New Risks

Technology has encouraged the proliferation of unverified new tests. Poorly verified tests are added without much study and without a suitable data base indicating their usefulness. The following example illustrating the potential misuse of a powerful technology in screening is hypothetical, but it follows a familiar format. Computer Axial Tomography (CAT scan) is a diagnostic technique of great value in some specific patients, and its inventors have been awarded the Nobel Prize in medicine. It has such high resolution that it can detect abnormal spots in the lung not seen on routine chest x-rays. What it cannot do is determine either the nature of these abnormal spots or their significance. The exact percentage of false positives that result from use of the CAT scan to detect lung cancer is not known, but it is estimated to be considerable.

Let us imagine that CAT scan is adopted as a screening procedure for normal subjects. It is used on a 45-year-old executive with a history of smoking two packs of cigarettes a day for 25 years. A small round spot, a nodule, is detected in the lung. One possible diagnosis is cancer of the lung, and, indeed, because of his smoking history, the executive is at increased risk of cancer of the lung. If this is the diagnosis, and if it is accurate, then the cancer has been detected at a time when the prognosis for cure by surgery might be most favorable. The fact is that many small nodules in the lungs of smokers are not cancer; however, once the nodule has been detected by a CAT scan, the patient will be subjected to a series of tests. His sputum will be examined for cancer cells. If cancer cells are found in the sputum, it means that lung cancer is present; but even repeated negative results of sputum examinations do not rule out cancer. Let us say that no cancer cells are found.

Now the patient undergoes a bronchoscopy: The doctor pushes a tube into the bronchial tubes—under either local or general anesthesia—and searches for cancer tissue. Even if cancer is present, when the nodules are small the test is usually negative; but it is reliable only when positive. In this instance, the result is negative. The next step may be an attempt to put a needle through the chest wall to obtain tissue from the nodule itself. Again, the test is negative. But again, this does not rule out cancer, and an open-lung biopsy follows. This, you may remember, is a major surgical procedure in which the chest is opened and tissue obtained directly from the lung. When the lungs are visualized directly, there may be no nodule. All of these studies may have been dictated by phantom shadows picked up by the CAT scan and cast by nonexistent nodules; its tendency to do just this constitutes a limitation of the technique.

It may well be that a huge number of normal subjects will show nodules on CAT scanning, as did our hypothetical patient, but in only a few instances can they, or do they need to be, treated. New techniques, because of their high resolution, show up large numbers of false-positive findings. In fact, the number may be so large that to operate on all of them is impractical, in which case a patient would be told, "You have a nodule in your lung—it may be cancer or it may not be cancer, we don't know. What we will do is have you come in every three months and we'll continue to observe the lesion by repeated CAT scans. If the nodule becomes larger, we'll operate; if not, then we'll just watch it." Now the doctor puts his arm around the shoulder of the patient and says, "Go home and don't worry." Finally, repeated exposure to x-rays during CAT scanning could cause cancer of the lung; the patient may ultimately develop a cancer of the lung because he has been subjected to the original test.

If you re-read this section, you will see that a trick has been played on you. Our 45-year-old executive was first identified as a subject. Once the CAT scan was performed, he became a patient. This could easily happen, and with potentially tragic results.

This example is hypothetical but not farfetched in its implications. It indicates that advances in medical technology may create new hazards—and that the minimal requirement for introducing a new test should be to verify its usefulness in a small representative population before applying it broadly.

Verification should be the responsibility of the doctors *introducing* the test and not of those who *challenge* it. It also illustrates the potentially devastating effect of a false-positive result and indicates that a test may be appropriate for individuals with actual disease but quite inappropriate as a test for apparently normal people. It supports our contention that the risks and benefits should be known *before* and not after the introduction of the test.

Executive Health Program

Periodic health examinations continue to flourish. A favored form is the executive health program, in which a company provides these examinations at no cost to its top executives. Perhaps this serves as a form of revenge for the inadequate health resources that many of the poor command. Who knows, perhaps "blessed are the poor" because they are not subjected to the needless health testing of the rich. There has been little attempt to eliminate tests demonstrably ineffective in improving health care, such as routine electrocardiograms. Moreover, as new tests or new technologies appear, they tend to be incorporated quickly into the routine examination. All of this goes on without any real attempt at risk-benefit analysis.

Multiphasic Screening

A variant of the annual physical examination is so-called multiphasic screening, a series of studies that focuses on laboratory tests and is usually offered by huge health care establishments. Tests may include an electro-cardiogram; measurements of lung function and blood pressure; a hearing test; chest, abdominal, and bone x-rays; mammography; measurements of vision and pressure within the eye; measurements of height, weight, and thickness of skin; a general physical examination; gynecological examination, Pap smears, and breast examination; a self-administered questionnaire concerning health and psychological status; and sigmoidoscopy. There is no evidence to suggest that, on the whole, the medical benefits derived from this huge battery of tests outweigh the risks. For the owners of the clinics offering the tests, however, the economic benefits are enormous.

Some Useful Surveys

As a relief from this dreary picture, let us consider two forms of health surveys that are almost certainly useful.

Periodic Examinations of Healthy Children

One of the benefits of the periodic examination of normal children is that it creates the opportunity to administer vaccines for immunizing children against whooping cough, diphtheria, measles, mumps, tetanus, and poliomyelitis. Careful studies have shown that such immunization programs pay major health dividends—but they could be administered in settings other than periodic health examinations. There are, inevitably, risks; both whooping-cough vaccine and measles vaccine may be associated with encephalitis. But, on balance, the risk-benefit ratio seems to be sharply favorable for children who are vaccinated.

Periodic examination of children also appears to be useful in detecting a variety of treatable diseases. Theoretically, a comparison of the physical development of the individual child (height, weight, etc.) with the range of normal values permits the detection of nutritional problems, of various disease states such as kidney disease and congenital heart disease, and evidence of child abuse. Finally, the pediatrician can provide emotional support to parents newly confronted with the problems of raising a child.

Many pediatricians pride themselves on limiting the number of studies they pursue in well children, and perhaps that accounts for the generally favorable attitude toward this form of periodic examination.

Periodic Prenatal Examinations

Expectant mothers are another group of patients who can benefit by periodic examinations. The physician can, for example, take preventive measures against Rh disease. A result of incompatibility of blood groups between mother and fetus, Rh disease often causes the death of the fetus or newborn child. Injections of Rh immune globulin, a protein found in plasma, given at the time of birth to Rh negative women with Rh positive husbands, will prevent the disease. The effectiveness of this treatment has been documented by properly conducted clinical trials.

A number of diseases peculiar to pregnancy, or worsened by pregnancy, can be detected and treated. Because these illnesses are usually limited to pregnancy and the postnatal period, this form of periodic examination makes sense, but there are risks. Overtesting of the pregnant patient may lead to the same complications as those that arise in other forms of periodic health examinations—but two lives are at stake. For example, a routine ultrasound examination of the uterus has been proposed. Not only is there some question about the safety of this procedure for the fetus, but the frequency and consequences of false positives are unknown. A dramatic example of a false-positive ultrasound test is recounted in Chapter 8. In general, the risk-benefit ratio for prenatal examination appears to be favorable, perhaps because of the special circumstances surrounding pregnancy.

Tests on the Newborn

Three tests have a substantial positive impact on the health of newborns. Congenital hypothyroidism, caused by a lack of thyroid hormone, is a disease in which untreated children develop severe permanent mental retardation; it occurs in about one in every 4,000 births. The detection of hypothyroidism by appropriate testing in the newborn is relatively simple and reasonably accurate. Treatment with thyroid hormone is highly effective in preventing mental retardation and has a lifelong beneficial effect.

Phenylketonuria (PKU), a rare inherited disorder, also results in mental retardation when untreated. It can be successfully treated by restricting the subject to a simple diet throughout most of childhood. The treatment is eminently practical— the special diet can be discontinued at a relatively early age, but the treated subject remains normal throughout life. The screening test is relatively simple and accurate; even if it were to produce a false positive, the child would not be harmed. The dietary treatment has no dire consequences and does not adversely affect lifestyle. Mental retardation due to PKU has been virtually eradicated in the United States and Great Britain.

Galactosemia is a disorder attributable to an inherited deficiency of an enzyme specifically required for the normal metabolism of certain sugars—galactose and lactose—in the body. The sugar accumulates in the brain, the liver, the kidney, and the lens of the eye; mental retardation, cataracts, and abnormalities of liver and kidney function follow. The disease can be detected by a test performed on the red blood cells of newborns. Treated with a diet free of galactose or lactose, affected infants develop normally. The special diet would not impose a major hardship on a false positive. These three tests in newborns are impressive examples of the good that medicine does.

Cancer Screening of Normal Subjects

Cancer exacts a frightful toll in suffering and death in patients of almost every age group. Approximately 450,000 patients die of cancer each year in the United States.

Screening tests to detect cancer in normal subjects were introduced with the laudable goal of decreasing this carnage. The rationale underlying the use of screening tests at their inception reflected the best scientific information available at the time. The major mechanism of death from cancer was known to be metastasis, a spreading from the original site. The consensus was that early detection leading to early removal would be associated with an improved rate of salvage. It seemed logical that the earlier the detection, the smaller the original tumor would be and the less likely it would be to metastasize.

The increase in scientific knowledge of cancer since the introduction of cancer screening complicates, rather than simplifies, an evaluation of the usefulness of screening methods for early detection. Cancer arises from subtle change in perhaps a single cell. At this stage cancer is premalignant and its removal might result in a 100 percent cure rate. But many of these premalignant cells never go on to produce cancer. Screening methods, such as Pap smears, to detect early stages would result in surgical or other forms of treatment in a number of patients who never would have developed cancer— because the early malignant cells would not have developed into invasive cancer—and for whom treatment was not necessary.

Another complicating factor is that metastasis seems to depend on certain clones of cancer cells that are present early in the development of the disease. In some forms of cancer—oat cell cancer of the lung, for example—there appears to be spread of the cancer in the earliest stages, even before detection is possible. Surgical removal of the cancer is therefore not particularly helpful and a systemic form of cancer treatment, chemotherapy, is used.

As a consequence of the metastasizing clones, it may be that at the time of detection by a screening test—for instance, seeing a nodule on x-ray or detecting bleeding in the stool—

some cancers, even if small, are already far advanced, and the outcome for the patient is determined by factors largely independent of early detection and early treatment. In another kind of cancer, cancer of the prostate, metastasis takes place quite late or perhaps never. It is said that some very large percent of males over the age of 70—10 to 40 percent—have cancer of the prostate, and relatively few show metastatic disease. For this kind of cancer, in which metastasis is relatively rare, early detection by screening might not be useful.

No one would argue that removing an established cancer is not in most instances worthwhile. But it appears that the number of subjects who can potentially be helped by screening for early detection is significantly lower than originally believed. Cancer screening was introduced and has been applied to millions of patients, usually without adequate clinical trials. This raises the issue of what constitutes adequate evidence to establish the usefulness of a screening test—in my opinion, not the indirect and inferential evidence cited by most experts.

A few medical scientists have suggested that to continue to screen without adequate trials is to expose huge numbers of subjects to significant risks. But their protests are lost in an almost universal acceptance of current practice. In particular, the number and fate of false-positive patients have been virtually unexplored.

What accounts for this neglect? One distinguished cancer expert cites the enormous pressure to translate the results of laboratory studies into clinical practice during the early days of cancer screening—even though the evidence to support the usefulness of that translation was not available. Less charitable observers have suggested that expanded use of screening can be attributed to the economic, social, and political gains it has brought to its practitioners.

Wherever the responsibility lies, the use of cancer screening in normals is not based on rigorous standards. National or international organizations may endorse a given form of screening; official government bodies may endorse a given form of screening; learned experts may endorse it—none of these endorsements is based on the kind of evidence appropriate for an undertaking that has such important consequences for huge numbers of patients. This state of affairs might be acceptable if cancer screening conferred only benefits and was free of risks. You have learned that this is sadly not true.

Two Modern Diseases

At least partially as a result of the publicity surrounding cancer screening, two diseases have flourished in this country:

- *Cancerphobia,* a pathologic fear of cancer that so dominates the subject's life that he is distracted from leading a normal life.
- *Cancerguiltia,* a pathologic feeling of guilt when the subject or a family member develops cancer. A contributing factor to this disease is the tone some campaigns adopt to stimulate participation in cancer screening. The campaigns imply that the calamity is the fault of the patient or the family, because he could have avoided the disease by participating in the suggested test. Some campaigns explicitly state that this is the case.

Breast Self-Examination (BSE)

An unusually lucid and honest article written by an expert doctor for other doctors provides an opportunity to illustrate some of the problems associated with cancer screening. The author states that 75 to 90 percent of breast cancers are discovered by patients themselves, usually by accident. It therefore seems reasonable to assume that breast self-examination might lead to earlier detection, and earlier detection could result in a higher cure rate.

She states that "the real value of breast self-examination

could only be ascertained by studies showing that women randomly selected to be taught BSE—who learned how to perform it well—experienced lower breast cancer mortality than randomly selected controls who did not perform BSE. Such a study is impossible."

Two errors are apparent. The suggestion ignores women who are false positives and come to harm as a result of BSE. To be valid, any study would have to include their fate. No cogent reasons are advanced to establish that an adequate clinical trial is impossible. In fact, such a study could have been done and should have been done before BSE was introduced on a mass scale. That study could still be done.

The author describes the advantages of BSE: It is not invasive, costs nothing, is convenient, and can be done frequently. "Perhaps the strongest point in its favor," she notes, "is its high level of acceptability in the eyes of the general public, medical professionals and national cancer societies." This is an advantage from the standpoint of those promoting BSE, but it confers no direct medical benefits on participating subjects.

How about the disadvantages? "Much more numerous than the advantages, however, are the disadvantages." She describes several: BSE is associated with fear and anxiety. Women are uncertain about the nature of the abnormalities they are looking for. It may lead to unnecessary visits to doctors and generate unnecessary expenses. Large numbers of negative biopsies (self-examination has resulted in false positives) may result. All this may create a backlash. "Women with lumps which turn out to be false alarms may abandon self-examinations, while others may become too complacent and decide that a lesion is harmless, when it is not."

That women rarely perform the test adequately the author identifies as a major problem. In one study, one year after women were taught BSE on a one-to-one basis, no more than 2 to 3 percent of the students did an "ideal" examination.

Finally, the expert acknowledges, BSE seemed more acceptable to younger women than to older women, although the older women are at increased risk of breast cancer. She hopes that the younger women will persevere as they become older but does not suggest a rational basis for this hope. The article offers evidence that BSE results in detection of smaller and earlier cancers than those uncovered by accident but offers no data to establish that this produces a more favorable outcome.*

This article appeared in March of 1984. Obviously nothing had changed since 1978, when another expert, troubled by the same issues, wrote: "No matter how much its appeal we must insist on some sort of evidence before we set millions of women nervously palpating their breasts in front of a mirror every month in response to subway advertisements, cancer society commercials, television, and books published for the lay public."

Breast self-examination is an appealing, widely accepted, and intensively touted test whose risks and benefits have not been determined and are in fact largely unknown. Women should not be urged to participate until such information is available.

Papanicolaou (Pap) Smear

As you read this section of the book you should be aware that many excellent organizations such as the American Cancer Society, the National Cancer Institute, and a variety of international groups endorse periodic or annual Pap smears for cervical cancer. These groups receive advice from some of the world's leading cancer experts, but neither the opinions of the numerous societies nor of the experts are based on any *acceptable* prospective clinical trial of the risks versus benefits of Pap smear. I am not an expert in uterine cancer, but the facts are as I have stated them.

*Reprinted with permission, Cornelia J. Baines, "Breast Self-Examination: The Doctor's Role," *Hospital Practice,* vol. 19, no. 4 (March 1984): 120.

One of the most widely used tests in medical history, the regular or annual cervical Pap smear is used to detect early cancer of the uterine cervix. Superficial cells scraped from the cervix are stained by a technique introduced by an American doctor (for whom the test is named, George Nicolas Papanicolaou), and examined under the microscope.

An astronomical number of women undergo this study. In 1976, approximately 60 percent of American women 18 to 34 years of age reported having had a Pap test the previous year; 82 percent reported having had at least one Pap test during a lifetime. This remarkable rate of participation is in part attributable to effective publicity campaigns to convince women of the importance of annual Pap smears: 1957 was designated as "Uterine Cancer Year" and in the 1970s we had the "Let No Woman Be Overlooked" program. Despite all the publicity, cancer of the cervix is not a common cause of death.

The routine use of the test in apparently normal women has even been endorsed in a court decision: A doctor suggested on several occasions that a patient undergo cervical Pap testing. The patient did not accept the suggestion. She ultimately died of cervical cancer, and her family successfully sued the doctor and collected a substantial sum of money on the grounds that the doctor had not provided the patient sufficient information to enable her to exercise the right of informed refusal. This meant presumably that the risks and benefits of the test were not adequately explained.

Most women believe in the value of the Pap smear, as do most doctors. But the factors to be considered are more complex than the screened population and many doctors appreciate. Actually, substantial risks as well as benefits are attached to the test. The truth is that there has never been an acceptable study either to confirm the value of the Pap test in apparently normal women or to indicate the magnitude of the risks. Despite this, it has been and is used on millions of women.

Evidence is cited for the efficacy of cervical Pap smears in prolonging life. It is claimed that:

- Cervical screening can identify women who are at greater than average risk of developing invasive cervical cancer.
- The widespread use of screening has been accompanied by substantial reductions in the incidence of cervical cancer and in the death rate from this disease.
- Therapy based on positive smears can reduce the incidence and mortality rates of invasive cervical cancer; this is shown by *(a)* declining rates in centers with increasing rates before screening was instituted, and *(b)* lower rates among screened women than among unscreened women. (Death from cervical cancer has also declined in regions where few or no women are screened, but this is largely ignored.)

The evidence indicating the benefits of Pap smears is derived from studies that were not controlled and is without supporting data on the number and the fate of false positives. Many experts find this evidence acceptable, but even some of them are uneasy at the disparity between the inadequate nature of the evidence and the enormous number of women who are screened.

The Risk of a False Positive

Here is one woman's experience: Healthy and in her 40s, she undergoes a Pap test; it is reported positive and several more are performed. A diagnosis of cancer of the cervix is made and she is told that surgery will be needed. She is advised that she requires a total hysterectomy plus removal of the ovaries. This advice produces intense emotional turmoil. Her husband asks the patient's doctor how often false-positive Pap smears occur. He does not receive a satisfactory answer but has the impression that he and his wife are being told that this seldom or never happens. Dissatisfied, they refer themselves to a leading cancer hospital. The husband pursues the question of how often false-positive Pap smears occur and still does not obtain a clear answer.

A battery of tests, including more Pap smears, are performed at the second hospital and interpreted as showing no cancer. No operation is performed. The wife and husband are deeply resentful; had they been more passive, she would have undergone unnecessary surgery. They realize that no satisfactory answer to their question about false positives exists.

The facts concerning Pap smears are as follows. Experience suggests that the use of Pap smears in women who have manifestations suggesting cancer of the reproductive tract is valuable. For example, vaginal bleeding of unknown cause is sufficient indication for a Pap smear. This is a legitimate, well-documented, and valuable application of the Pap test.

About 40 years ago, the use of Pap testing was extended to normal women for the purpose of early detection of cervical cancer. The rationale for this extension was as follows: Cancer of the cervix develops from a single abnormal cancer cell or nests of cancer cells. For a period of time, these cancer cells remain localized; this form of cancer or precancer is known as carcinoma in situ (CIS) and does not produce symptoms. Theoretically, removing cancer at this stage should cure the disease.

Usually, after many (perhaps 10 to 35) years, the cancer cells become invasive, a condition known as invasive carcinoma of the cervix (ICC). At this point, the cancer becomes symptomatic and spreads, first within the uterus and finally to other organs and structures. This process of invasion usually takes months to years. Removal of the cancer in the localized state (CIS) is associated with high cure rates, perhaps 100 percent. Removal of the cancer after it is invasive is less likely to be curative.

Difficulties in Interpretation

The cervical Pap smear was introduced as a method for detecting the earliest possible stage of cancer and thereby improving the chances for cure. It was advocated as an annual examination so that each woman would go no more than one year with an undetected cancer. That is the theory. The practice is not so simple. First of all, Pap smears require interpretation, but it is often difficult to determine whether or not cancer cells are present; various doctors examining the same specimen under the microscope will vary widely in their opinions. In one study, there was disagreement among 10 experts as to the presence or absence of cancer cells in about 40 percent of the specimens. In another study, in about two-thirds of the subjects, two Pap smears taken simultaneously from the same woman showed different results—no cancer in one sample and cancer in the other.

A noncancerous alteration called dysplasia occurs in the cells of the cervix and may be difficult or impossible to distinguish from CIS. Abnormal cells appear in the Pap smear as a result of various causes—fungal infections, changes in metabolic state of the subject, or for reasons not yet determined. The possibility of finding in the Pap smear abnormal noncancerous cells that can be mistaken for cancer is substantial. Abnormal Pap smears are classified into five categories, and only one, class 5 cells, shows ICC.

Not uncommonly, when a uterus is removed after a series of abnormal Pap smears no evidence of cancer is found despite careful examination (false positive). Conversely, women have been found to have ICC shortly after a negative Pap smear. Thus, a significant number of false negatives must exist.

The evidence indicates an unknown but very high percentage of false-positive Pap smears—false positive because of false interpretation; false positive in the sense that the patient would not have developed ICC even if the CIS had not been treated; false positive in the sense that no CIS may be found after removal of the uterus; and false positive in the sense that a number of other factors such as infection result in cervical cells that look like CIS. There is some evidence that certain kinds of cervical infections and dysplastic changes can ultimately lead to cancer. The evidence is convincing to some doctors but not to others.

How much good has the massive use of Pap smears accomplished? It is difficult to estimate. There has been a decline in death rates from ICC, some—perhaps most, but not all—of which can be attributed to the mass use of cervical Pap smears. Undoubtedly, many individual patients have benefited from the procedure.

How much harm has the mass use of Pap smears done? Again, this is difficult to estimate; probably a large amount, judging from the high incidence of false-positive results. The extent of the harm depends on what is done to false-positive patients in the mistaken belief that they have cancer. The worst outcome is that they die during unnecessary surgery. In abdominal or vaginal hysterectomy—removal of the uterus—the death rate from surgery is approximately 2 deaths per 1,000 operations.

The impact of surgery is even more sharply unfavorable for the false-positive subject than the simple mortality figures indicate. How many years of life are saved by early detection of cancer by a Pap smear? ICC takes many years to develop from CIS, and after the disease develops it usually takes several more years before the patient succumbs. Operative and postoperative deaths from hysterectomy occur quickly. If a true-positive CIS is present at age 35 and not treated, the patient, assuming the ultimate development of ICC, will on the average not die for perhaps 30 years. Life expectancy is now about 75 years for American women. Therefore, the years of life saved by the test would be 75 minus 65, or 10 years. The test would add 10 woman-years of survival for each case of early detection by the test.

Death from hysterectomy results quickly, either at surgery or within days to weeks after the operation. A 35-year-old woman with a false-positive test who dies of surgery might lose 40 years (75 minus 35). To achieve a balance, three to four times the number of woman-years lost because of surgery would have to be saved by early detection. Neither I nor anyone else knows the actual figures for either years saved or years lost, but the risk of premature and needless death is real.

Hysterectomy results in about 350 significant complications per 1,000 operations. This must be counted as a real risk of a false-positive Pap smear. A number of false-positive patients are managed, not with hysterectomy, but with other forms of treatment. Essentially all false-positive patients go through emotional and psychological trauma. Even without precise statistics, we can be certain that large numbers of normal subjects have been harmed by Pap testing.

Alternatives to Hysterectomy

No single acceptable approach to managing normal subjects with abnormal Pap smears is universally accepted. One approach is to do a second series of Pap tests as soon as the first abnormality is detected. Even if subsequent smears prove negative, the patient undergoes periodic Pap tests—now, not as a normal person, but as a cancer suspect.

Periodic colposcopy is increasingly used; in this test the cervix is examined with a magnifying lens. If abnormal areas in the cervix are found, a biopsy of the cervix is done.

Still another approach is to perform a diagnostic biopsy of the cervix. Abnormal areas on the cervix are identified by painting the cervix with an iodine solution; cancerous areas do not take up the iodine solution but stand out as white areas, and a section of the white area is biopsied. This is known as the Shiller test. Despite its former widespread use, the test is so nonspecific that it has been largely abandoned.

Diagnostic conization is another test frequently used. In this, a cone of cervix is removed for a biopsy.

Each of these tests has its limitations in terms of sensitivity, specificity, and accuracy. Some may be harmful. For example, the rate of complication with conization is said to be about 10 percent and includes postconization hemorrhage, infection, cervical stenosis (narrowing of the cervix by scar), and infertility.

There are several approaches to treatment of CIS. Hysterectomy is the most radical and almost certainly the most common form of treatment. Suspicious areas of the cervix may be removed by freezing the affected area (cryosurgery), by laser surgery, or by therapeutic conization. Radiation treatment may also be used. Each of these treatments has an inherent morbidity and mortality.

Experts disagree on therapy for dysplasia. Some experts believe that severe dysplasia should be treated like cancer. Others believe that mild to moderate dysplasia should be treated like cancer. Others disagree with both these opinions.

No general agreement has been reached on follow-up for patients with moderately suspicious Pap smears. It is possible for an apparently normal 25-year-old female who shows a class 3 Pap smear, consistent with mild to moderate dysplasia, to be followed as a cancer suspect for the remaining 50 years of her life. What, for example, should she tell a prospective husband? You can imagine the impact on the quality of her life.

These uncertainties of management are no different in the normal subject with an abnormal Pap smear than in patients with manifestations of cervical disease. But two critical differences do exist between the two groups: First, the incidence of false positives is much lower in patients who show manifestations; the patient with symptoms of cervical disease is ʰy definition at a higher risk for cancer than the normal subject. Second, the patient with cervical disease consulted a doctor because of explicit symptoms. The normal subject had no symptoms but came for a Pap smear because it was recommended; she was unaware of the possibility of a false-positive finding and the ensuing consequences.

Weighing the Risks and Benefits

Are there more risks than benefits? The truth is that no one knows. The use of the test has never been studied in an *adequate* prospective clinical trial, so that an accurate estimate of risks and benefits is not available. It is possible that, on balance, the use of Pap smears has resulted in more harm than good to women. It is also possible that its use has resulted in more good than harm.

Would it be feasible to remedy the situation by conducting a clinical trial so that women might be offered the test as an informed and rational choice? The answer is almost certainly not. Most authorities who sponsor mass testing of this type claim that such a trial would be "unethical." In medicine this appeal to ethics is usually evoked when the evidence for the effectiveness of a given intervention is so overwhelming that depriving the patient of the intervention will clearly harm her. This is simply not true of the Pap test.

Organizing a clinical trial at this time would, however, be almost impossible because of the difficulty of enlisting volunteers to act as controls—the controls would not undergo regular Pap smears—and other volunteers who would agree to go through the inconveniences a trial would require.

You might want to pause a few minutes and analyze your reaction to this part of the book. If you are a man, you probably have not been deeply concerned with the issues. If you are a woman, you may be thinking that what you have just read simply cannot be true. All your previous experience leads you to believe that your doctors and the medical profession could not have subjected masses of women to an unproven and potentially harmful test. You just know that the Pap test is reliable. Your reaction may even cause you to wonder whether the rest of this book is as balanced as it should be.

Recall that Pap smears in this country were originally recommended as an annual test. In 1979, this policy was modified; now "regular" rather than annual Pap smears are recommended by one influential organization. Other advice is provided by other groups. The National Cancer Institute, a government agency, suggests that all sexually active women should have a minimum of three examinations over a period

of years. Some Institute scientists still believe in annual examinations; others believe that an examination once every three
years is adequate. A task force of the Canadian government
has still another series of recommendations. Other groups
have still other opinions. In practice, some doctors continue
to advise annual Paps; others follow the recommendations of
one organization or another. What this should tell you is that
no one really knows, because the data base for a precise
recommendation is simply not available.

The use of cervical Paps in apparently normal women was
introduced at a time when the importance of adequate prospective clinical trials was not recognized. The use of the test
has now become so established that it is doubtful, as I have
explained, that such a trial could be conducted at this time.
Much could be done, however, to determine its usefulness and
to decrease its risks.

A national study could be undertaken to determine just how
reproducible interpretations of Pap smears are. An organized
national effort could be made to find women who have not
been Pap tested and then to determine the incidence and
mortality of cervical cancer in this untested group. The various
diagnostic and therapeutic measures used to manage women
with abnormal Pap smears could be evaluated by clinical trials.
None of these would adequately substitute for a prospective
clinical trial of cervical Pap testing, but each would provide
critically important information not currently available.

How should you, as a woman, make a decision about Pap
smears? At the very least, be as sure as you can that you are
not a false positive. Do not assume that your doctor necessarily
knows more about the limitations of the test than you do. In
fact, having read this section, you may know more about the
problems than your doctor does. And do not let your doctor
be in too much of a hurry to remove your uterus. If you decide
against annual Pap smears or even a regular schedule of Pap
smears, do not feel guilty. Lend your support to efforts in
medicine to gather accurate clinical information before the

introduction and mass application of practices with far-reaching consequences.

Mammography

Cancer of the breast, unlike cancer of the cervix, is a major cause of death and disability in the United States. It reportedly claims the lives of 35,000 to 40,000 women each year. Vigorous attempts to reduce this high death rate are obviously indicated.

Yearly screening for cancer by mammography of the breast for women aged 35 to 70 was first advocated in the United States in 1973. Major support for the recommendation was based on a limited clinical trial conducted in New York City during the 1960s. Some 62,000 women aged 40 to 70 were randomly divided into two groups of equal size. One group (the study group) was offered annual mammography and physical examination; the second (control) group was merely observed. There was only a small difference between the two groups. Interestingly, of the 299 breast cancers found in the study group, only 132, less than half, were detected by mammography alone. After ten years, however, cancer deaths were significantly though not dramatically lower in the study group. Ninety-three women died in the study group, whereas 133 women died in the control group. This difference, extrapolated to millions of women, suggests the possibility of a major improvement in outcome. There was evidence that women at high risk for the development of breast cancer tended to self-select for screening. If so, then the results would be more favorable than might be expected from screening all women.

Although too limited in scope and number, this study represented an important beginning. Careful analysis of the data, however, revealed that mammography made no significant difference in survival in women under the age of 50. Despite these limitations, mass annual screening of women was introduced in the United States for women aged 35 or older. Three years later, the recommendation was modified to apply only to women aged 50 or older. This change was not prompted by any new information; it came about because the experts began to worry about one of the three important risks associated with mammography—that the cumulative x-ray doses associated with its use could cause cancer of the breast.

Expert opinion ranged from assurances that the risk of induced cancer was trivial to the statement that "[it is] regretfully concluded that there seems to be a possibility that the routine use of mammography in screening asymptomatic women may eventually take almost as many lives as it saves." Other evidence surfaced. One hundred and twenty of a group of 1,800 women with breast masses considered to be cancer of the breast turned out, upon review, to have no cancer or questionable cancer. Most of these underwent radical mastectomy—some, most, or all, unnecessarily. The original decision to mammogram indiscriminately was unquestionably, as stated by one cancer authority, characterized by "a general pattern of single-minded pursuit of breast cancer detection to the exclusion of such relevant considerations as false-positive results, radiation hazards, the cost of the procedure and the evidence of effectiveness."

Shifting Recommendations

The new recommendations, in 1976, were that women between the ages of 35 to 40 have a baseline mammogram and women over 50 have a mammogram each year. The uncertainty that underlies these shifts in opinion is sharply illustrated by the contrast in the following examples. A 45-year-old woman switched gynecologists. Her first gynecologist did not believe in mammography; consequently, she had no mammograms. The second refused to act as her doctor unless she submitted to mammograms. She reluctantly agreed and her mammogram revealed a breast mass. She underwent a biopsy, the mass was cancerous and surgically removed. Nothing will ever persuade her or her gynecologist that mammography is not a valuable contribution to the welfare of patients.

A 57-year-old woman, without evidence of cancer, underwent routine mammography. A mass in the left breast was discovered. She was hospitalized in a state of extreme anxiety and told that if the biopsy were positive, the surgeon would perform a radical mastectomy. The biopsy did not reveal cancer of the breast. She does not know whether or not to subject herself to future mammograms.

In 1983, a new set of recommendations was offered. With great fanfare, it was announced that the yearly mammogram should be employed in women aged 40 or older. Again, the change was not based on new data but on new technology and a shift in the attitude of doctors concerning treatment for cancer of the breast. The new technology reduces the dose of radiation required to provide satisfactory mammograms to approximately one-third the dose delivered in the 1970's. It is reasonable to assume that the smaller dose of radiation would cause less cancer, or perhaps not cause cancer at all. The shift in medical attitude is the acceptance of lumpectomy and radiation as effective treatment for patients with small cancers at the time of diagnosis (see Chapter 8). With the adoption of new and less devastating treatment it appeared more useful to attempt early detection of lesions. These assumptions are implicit in this recommendation.

You may be interested to know how the change in recommendation was brought about. Some months before, a committee of experts had met and recommended that the policy of yearly mammograms restricted to women over age 50 and women at high risk for cancer of the breast be maintained. The vote was exceedingly close, indicating that, at best, any change was controversial. Some months later the same committee met, but with minor changes in its composition. The vote was again exceedingly close, but this time a bare majority voted to include women aged 40 and older in routine mammography.

The experts transmitted none of their doubts or disagreements to the public. The new policy was announced with great public hoopla, and the process of selling the new policy to millions of women in the 40 to 50 age group started. Had the experts publicized the dubious as well as the positive aspects, they would have enabled women to make a more informed decision.

Experts at the National Cancer Institute have been more cautious. The Institute has issued a statement that there is "suggestive evidence, but no solid proof that mammography benefits now outweigh the risks." One official stated, "I'd rather await completion of a study in Canada that should provide further evidence."

Risks of the Annual Mammogram

What are the risks of yearly mammograms? One is the risk of cancer from exposure to radiation. The relatively low doses now employed have presumably lessened this risk. By how much? This is not known; no one has data precise enough to make possible an accurate calculation of the risk of cancer.

The second risk is that of creating false-positive patients. This outcome creates needless emotional trauma for every patient. It also leads to an unnecessary biopsy of the breast, not a formidable surgical procedure, but not a trivial one either. While not as life-threatening as hysterectomy, breast biopsy does have its own intrinsic morbidity and mortality. How common are false-positive mammograms? Evidence suggests that for every cancer uncovered, five to ten biopsies performed on the basis of a positive mammogram turn out to be noncancerous. This means that perhaps ten operations are required to detect a single case of cancer. This is not a happy ratio and it is clear that mammography is not a very specific procedure.

The third risk is that some cancers detected by mammography would not have required surgery at all. The true magnitude of the risk is not known, but one retrospective analysis suggested that one-third of the cancers detected by mammography fall into this category.

Now might be an opportune time to prevent a repetition of the Pap smear dilemma. A controlled study could be set up using 40-year-old women, who several months ago were advised to wait until age 50 to begin their annual mammograms. It should be possible to recruit enough volunteers to serve as controls in a situation where the best that can be offered to women generally is unknown. Those who argue against waiting for adequate data could go ahead and urge mammograms for women not participating in the clinical trial.

What should you, as a prospective subject for periodic mammography, do? If you decide to participate, you run a substantial risk of undergoing unnecessary surgery, emotional trauma, and a small, but unknown, risk of possible radiation effects. You may decide to accept these risks but at least your choice will be relatively informed.

Stool Guaiac Examination

Cancer of the colon and rectum is the second most common cancer in the United States. In 1979, approximately 114,000 new cases were discovered, and there are at present approximately half a million patients with this diagnosis. Over half of these people will die of the disease.

The stool guaiac test detects the presence of blood in the stool. Why not simply look at the stool and see whether it is bloody or not? Because blood in the stool may not be visible to the naked eye. The stool may be black in color because the blood has been chemically altered as it passes through the gut. Blood in the stool not recognizable to the naked eye is called occult or hidden blood, and the stool guaiac test can detect this form of bleeding in the gut.

Blood in the stool arises from many causes. Hemorrhoids

are a common cause of rectal bleeding. Even eating meat may cause a positive test. One of the important causes of a positive test is cancer of the rectum or bladder.

Interest in the use of this test has been stimulated by the fact that the test is simple, can be in part performed by the subject himself, and is perhaps sensitive in detecting early cancer. Another screening method, sigmoidoscopy, by which a tube inserted into the rectum is used to visualize the bowel wall, does not reach high enough to detect many cancers and has not been adequately tested as a screen for cancer.

It has been proposed that everyone near the age of 50 have a guaiac slide test once a year. The subject prepares stool samples on guaiac glass slides for three consecutive bowel movements. The reason for the multiple samples is that bleeding may be intermittent. To increase the accuracy of the test, a special meat-free, high-residue diet should be started at least twenty-four hours before the first stool specimen is collected and continued for the next three days. Vitamin C and aspirin should be avoided because they cause false positives.

Suppose the guaiac test is positive. That does not necessarily mean that the patient has colorectal cancer. In fact, the odds may be substantially against the possibility. What happens then?

One or more of several tests will be performed. These include a rectal examination, in which the doctor inserts a gloved finger into the rectum and feels for areas that may be cancerous. If he finds such an area he orders a biopsy. The patient may first undergo proctosigmoidoscopy; the doctor inspects the inside of the bowel visually through a lighted tube passed into the rectum and lower colon. If he discovers a growth, a small piece of tissue is removed for biopsy. The patient may also undergo fiberoptic colonoscopy. The colonoscope is a flexible instrument that allows the doctor to examine the entire length of the colon. Any suspicious areas are biopsied. The patient usually undergoes a barium enema; contrast material is passed into the rectum and colon, and these organs are x-rayed. A variety of other tests may be performed, depending on the creativity of the individual doctor.

A Review of the Data

In 1978, a careful review of the stool guaiac test, after examining current evidence, concluded.

> There are insufficient data to indicate that screening for colorectal cancer by stool occult blood testing reduces mortality from the disease in a screened population participating in clinical trials. More time is needed for the ongoing clinical trials to collect enough additional data for assessment of survival, benefit, and risk possibilities, and economic feasibility. Although it is recognized that decisions must sometimes be based on incomplete evidence, caution is advised in the development of recommendations about mass screening programs for colorectal cancer at this time. This caution is based on the absence of a clear demonstration of *(a)* improved survival rates in screened individuals with colon cancer or *(b)* a net margin of benefit to health in comparison with the costs and risks entailed in the further study of all positive occult blood reactions by barium enema examination, endoscopy, or both.
>
> Until more knowledge of the benefits and risks of screening for this cancer site is available, mass screening demonstration programs should not be initiated by the Division of Cancer Control and Rehabilitation, National Cancer Institute.
>
> The benefit-cost-risk indexes for stool occult blood testing cannot be determined at this time. In the light of present information, the uncontrolled application of the method outside of special evaluation studies may not represent a wise use of health care resources and may not be of benefit to the recipients.*

Fairly clear? Another item for further study must be added —the outcome of a false-positive test. The story is familiar. A false-positive test produces needless anguish. It leads to a series of uncomfortable and occasionally harmful interventions.

*From the Consensus Development Conference on Mass Screening for Colorectal Cancer sponsored by MCI/NIH, June 26–28, 1978.

A recent report concerning the value of chemotherapy in metastatic colorectal cancer gives one pause. The study showed that there was no benefit to the patients receiving chemotherapy and subjected to the significant risks of this form of treatment.

Now, what has changed since the negative review of the stool guaiac test by the experts in 1978 and its enthusiastic endorsement by a national organization? Nothing much in the way of new facts or data.

What should you do with respect to the stool guaiac test? One option is not to use it until better data become available and you can decide rationally whether it helps, is neutral, or, on balance, causes harm.

Blood Pressure

Screening for hypertension (high blood pressure) is universally advocated. Evidence shows that in many patients treatment of hypertension reduces the incidence of stroke, heart attacks, heart failure, and kidney failure—and other complications most likely to occur in subjects with marked elevation of blood pressure. Treatment is available for reducing the blood pressure. (Treatment for mild increases in blood pressure is controversial.) In the early stages of hypertension, before complications are evident, there are usually no symptoms. This fact favors mass surveys of blood pressure. Hypertension in a treatable phase can be detected only by periodic measurements, but most of the agents useful in treating hypertension produce unpleasant and occasionally serious side effects. This naturally tends to discourage patients from taking the drugs, so that patient compliance may be poor.

At one time, a diagnosis of hypertension led to a vast series of tests to determine its cause. It is now recognized that we cannot yet determine a demonstrable cause for hypertension in most patients, and this practice has been largely abandoned.

All things being equal, occasional measurement of your blood pressure, even when you are feeling well, is not a bad idea. It is no longer necessary to consult a doctor for blood pressure measurements—and this is a major advance. New equipment makes it possible to take the measurements in stores and other public places. Should you detect an increase in your blood pressure, you can then consult a doctor.

Tonometry

Glaucoma is a disease associated with an increase in intraocular pressure—pressure inside the eye. An estimated 15 patients per one million population go blind from glaucoma each year. Screening with tonometry for all asymptomatic adults is commonly recommended. Tonometry, a simple, painless measurement of intraocular pressure, takes about five minutes. Screening is recommended because early treatment may stop the progression of glaucoma to blindness.

Many of the assumptions underlying the proposal to screen, however, are either wrong or unproven. Most subjects with an elevated intraocular pressure do not have glaucoma. The actual number of patients with an abnormally high measurement who have glaucoma is less than 1 percent. As a result, 99 percent of subjects undergo needless worry and expense for a disease they do not have. The false-positive rate is very high.

Treatment of either elevated intraocular pressure or established glaucoma with conventional drugs has not been shown to produce clear-cut improvement; nor has early treatment been shown to halt the progression of glaucoma. Screening by tonometry is therefore of dubious value. The facts have not, however, decreased the use of this test, either as an isolated screening procedure, as part of a routine physical examination, or as part of a multiphasic screening.

The Major Risk of Surveys

The most pernicious risk attached to the various forms of health care intervention in normal subjects has not been directly described. Health care intervention produces a preoccupation with disease that detracts from the quality of life and is itself unhealthy. Illness is an unfortunate fact of life but is usually episodic in nature. Most people are fundamentally healthy for most of their lives. Most humans are not fragile and are not disease-ridden.

Medicine has been guilty not only of overestimating the potential benefits it can confer, but of overemphasizing the potential dangers of illness. Each separate constituency in medicine pressures people to worry about its specific area of disease, with the result that people waste much time in being tested for diseases that will never strike. We worry about cancer, stroke, heart attack, diabetes, arthritis, glaucoma, hepatitis, epilepsy, neurologic disease, obesity, anorexia, liver disease, lung disease, ulcers, constipation, diarrhea, insomnia, sleep apnea, and countless other disorders. We could spend most of our time being tested for this, that, or the other thing. Living an effective life requires that we place limits on these preoccupations.

This has been a long and complex chapter with a simple message: Many of the practices of modern medicine result in the conversion of normal, healthy people into patients.

With some notable exceptions, most of the medical interventions currently employed in normal subjects appear to have little favorable influence on health; many are untested and some are either harmful or have unacceptably high risks.

Remember that life is to be lived. It is far too short to be lived in a state of obsession with the possibility or the prevention of disease. Not only is an ounce of prevention not terribly effective; it can cause a pound or more of distraction. Perhaps Ben Franklin was right—"Nothing is more fatal to health than overcare of it."

13

The Patient as Experimental Subject

Medical research takes two forms—basic research and clinical research. *Basic research* investigates the mechanisms by which various biological processes, including disease, operate; it may address nonmedical as well as medical questions. The investigator may study parts of cells, whole cells, tissues, organs, or whole animals; healthy humans or patients. *Clinical research* studies disease processes directly; the models are the same as those studied in basic research—and the ideas often originate in basic research. Observation of patients or theoretical assumptions may also give rise to research ideas. Clinical research ultimately requires studies on human subjects; without it, medical progress would cease.

Basic Research

Many major medical breakthroughs have originated in basic research, although at times the original observations have been far removed from any discernible application to human disease. Not uncommonly, these revolutionary findings have come about by accident. Effective treatment for tuberculosis stemmed from a study of soil bacteria. Penicillin originated in a study of fungi contaminating the culture dishes in which bacteria were being grown. Poliomyelitis vaccine originated in studies of the effects of viruses on isolated monkey cells. Human organ transplantation evolved from an attempt to determine why certain animals grow new limbs when old ones are removed. Genetic engineering resulted from attempts to understand how genetic mechanisms work in bacteria and yeast.

No application to human welfare was anticipated when these studies were first pursued. Basic research is by definition a very inefficient process; untold numbers of poor, irrelevant, and unsuccessful studies must be supported in order to produce the rare breakthrough relevant to human disease. Without basic research, medical progress would halt; medicine would be frozen in its present unsatisfactory state.

Clinical Research

Studies performed on human subjects investigate issues ranging from trivial to crucial. There is great diversity; technical matters, procedural methods, diagnostic methods, therapeutic methods, and mechanisms of disease are all suitable areas for investigation in humans. The fundamental objectives may be to gain a greater understanding of disease process, to find better technological approaches to the study of disease, to determine the potential usefulness of new drugs, to test new methods of treatment, or any number of other disease-oriented aims.

It is a common misconception that individual patients are used as guinea pigs, especially in university-affiliated hospitals, which mount intensive research efforts. The large number of studies performed on patients fosters this notion. Overtesting is an accepted part of medical care; it is not necessarily done for research purposes. However misapplied these tests are—and we have discussed their use and abuse at length—the objective is not solely to learn more about science, but to learn more about the patient so that he or she may be helped.

A primary concern in any investigation in humans is the safety of the participants. Serious efforts are made to assure that human investigation will be as safe, effective, and useful as possible. But the safety of a new approach cannot be absolutely guaranteed. National guidelines have been established, and a local review committee usually monitors their application to a particular study. The committee asks: Does the proposed intervention present serious potential risks to patients? Are the necessary monitoring precautions available to pick up unexpected hazards? Is the project worthwhile? Has the patient been adequately informed of the risks involved, and has he or she given informed consent?

The system of committee review has important limitations. Colleagues of the investigator comprise the review committee; a committee of people who work at the same institution may arrive at a less critical evaluation than would a committee of outsiders. The committee completes its review and approves the study prior to its actual performance. It asks for annual reports of the study results; but once the study starts, periodic reviews may be perfunctory. As data are accumulated and hazards uncovered, patients may be subject to unanticipated risks. The quality of the proposed study may not be carefully assessed, and trivial topics are often approved. In these instances, patients are participating in a study that cannot add significantly to clinical knowledge. Despite their shortcomings, review committees do represent a forward step; there was a time when no reviews at all were required.

Human investigation, essential to medical progress, usually depends on the voluntary and altruistic participation of patients. Occasionally, doctors themselves provide striking examples of altruism and heroic behavior.

Idiopathic thrombocytopenia purpura (ITP) is a disease characterized by a dramatic decrease in the number of platelets in the blood; these cells are important in the process of clotting, and when this decrease takes place hemorrhaging in numerous organs of the body results. Some years ago, preliminary studies suggested that ITP might be caused by a chemical factor present in the plasma, the liquid part of the blood.

A young hematologist, fully aware of the potential risks,

decided to test this theory on himself. He obtained plasma from a patient afflicted with ITP and injected it into his own vein. The experiment proved successful; he became seriously ill. The number of platelets in his blood decreased dramatically, causing hemorrhages in various parts of his body. He survived, and his heroism made possible an important addition to the understanding of ITP.

A Disastrous Human Experiment

Let us consider a less laudable example. Coccidioidomycosis is a common fungal infection found primarily in the western part of the United States. It can affect many organs, including the lungs, skin, and, most seriously, the meninges, the membranes covering the brain. When the meninges are infected by the fungus, the disease is called coccidioidomycosis meningitis, or inflamed meninges. Coccidioidomycosis meningitis is associated with a substantial number of deaths, as well as short- and long-term disability.

A moderately effective drug for the treatment of coccidioidomycosis infection is amphotericin B. Although it is quite toxic, a risk-benefit analysis would indicate that it is the treatment of choice for serious coccidioidomycosis infections such as meningitis. Usually administered by vein, in meningitis it is often administered directly into the spinal fluid.

A derivative of this drug, amphotericin B methylester, was developed by a research chemist. Studied in animals, the new drug appeared to be relatively safe. The experts disagreed, however, about its potential value in the treatment of human coccidioidomycosis; some believed that the drug was one-fourth to one-eighth less toxic than amphotericin B, but also was one-fourth to one-eighth less effective as a treatment against the fungus. This meant that the larger doses of the new agent required for treatment would wipe out the advantage of less toxicity. Other experts believed that its decreased toxicity offered potential advantages.

A university hospital agreed to study the use of the drug in the treatment of human coccidioidomycosis meningitis. Formal requirements for human protection were met and the study was approved by the local human experimentation committee. Patients signed a form explaining the known dangers of the new drug and thus gave their "informed" consent to being used as subjects in the trial.

The drug was administered directly into the spinal fluid of a number of patients; several developed abnormal brain function and died. Death is not an unusual outcome in patients with this form of meningitis; however, a pathologist who examined the brains of the dead patients was convinced that the deaths could not be attributed to the fungal infection but rather to the use of the new drug, amphotericin B methylester. The principal investigator—the physician in charge of the study—strongly disagreed, arguing that abnormalities of brain tissue are common in patients dying of coccidioidomycosis, so that the deaths were not necessarily attributable to the new drug. The pathologist urged that the test be halted immediately; the principal investigator wanted it to continue.

The controversy exploded in the medical school community, in the news media, and, finally, in the law courts. While this was going on, the medical literature reported that brain damage had been found in patients who did not have coccidioidomycosis meningitis but who had been administered the new drug by vein, not into the spinal fluid.

The human experimentation committee at the university decided that the study must be terminated. The Food and Drug Administration (FDA) in Washington issued an edict that the drug not be used on human subjects. Meanwhile, the chemist who originally developed amphotericin B methylester discovered that the pharmaceutical company had added to the manufactured product some contaminating compounds not present in the original batch of the drug and capable of producing brain injury.

The problem did not end here. The principal investigator

was not able to use amphotericin B methylester at his own hospital. When consulted by physicians at other hospitals, however, he furnished the drug for their use. The matter was explored and he was found to be within his rights: The human experimentation committee had jurisdiction only at its own institution, and the FDA, believing further steps to be unnecessary, had not completed all of the formal requirements for withdrawing the drug from human use.

As a result, a toxic drug continued to be used in patients even after substantial questions had been raised about its safety. Most experts now believe that the new drug does produce brain injury. Some patients who participated in the study are currently suing for redress of injury—and some families for redress of death. The legal issues have yet to be settled.

As unusual and, thankfully, atypical as this example may be, it offers significant lessons: Subjects can and do die as a result of participating in research studies. In most studies, the risks of death are small and may be ignored; in some, the risks of death are unknown. Death does, however, represent the ultimate hazard to the human research subject. It is clear, too, that the results of animal studies do not necessarily apply to human subjects; in this case, the response of the animals studied did not provide clues to the disastrous effects the drug might have in humans. The example also shows the shortcomings of a review limited to the preliminary phase of a study. Unexpected hazards may not become apparent until months or years after a study is completed. In this instance, the pathologist fortunately sounded the alarm early in the study.

Guarding the Patient's Safety

New methods ultimately require testing in humans, but the present system of safeguarding human subjects does not always work. *Informed* consent was meant to be a safeguard for the patient, but under some circumstances truly informed consent is not possible. The patient is handed a written form that exhaustively describes the studies to be performed and lists the known risks. The investigator, or a representative of the investigator—or the patient's primary physician—adds an oral interpretation. But anyone who has seen critically ill patients with coccidioidomycosis meningitis will recognize that this is hardly a time when a patient can make rational decisions about complex matters. Many patients do not read the form carefully; beyond that, the language is often not easy to understand. In fact, the information is usually complex and often difficult for even trained medical people to grasp. At times legal information is included and an experienced attorney may be necessary to interpret the document.

Suppose the Golden Rule—Do unto others as you would have others do unto you—was applied, and a doctor suffering from coccidioidomycosis meningitis was asked, "Are you willing to try an experimental and untested new drug for the treatment of your dread disease?" Few, if any, would consent. The process for obtaining informed consent frequently assumes a degree of medical knowledge that few patients possess; and it further assumes an ability to apply this knowledge at a time when the patient may be too ill to make a reasonable judgment.

Conflicting Objectives

Research on patients raises another issue. The objectives of the investigator may conflict with those of the doctor responsible for the care of the patient. The researcher wants to obtain the most clear-cut answer to the issues under study; the patient's physician wants to achieve the best possible results for his patient. Often these interests coincide, but not invariably. For example, heart-lung transplantation has been cited in this book as an example of enlightened care on the part of a group of investigators. In order to obtain the clear answer they require as to the clinical usefulness of the procedure, investigators believe they must restrict their operations to patients free of other diseases.

On the basis of this criterion, a 39-year-old woman who had been operated on for cancer of the breast five years before was rejected when she applied for a heart-lung transplant. There was no evidence of recurrence of her cancer; she was a potential candidate for a heart-lung transplant because she had developed pulmonary hypertension. But it could not be determined beyond any doubt that she had been cured of cancer. The surgeon's decision was probably correct. To establish the effectiveness of what is still an experimental procedure, investigators studying heart-lung transplant are required to select the most suitable candidates. It would also have been entirely appropriate for her private physician to attempt to have her accepted for the surgery because it was her only chance for survival.

In the study of coccidioidomycosis, it appears that the zeal of the principal investigator may have blinded him to the harm suffered by some of the patients. When they began to do poorly, for whatever reason, it would have been prudent to stop the study. This would have handicapped the study, but would probably have been in the patients' best interests.

Frequently a given experimental procedure serves both the best interests of the patient and the needs of medical science. There are sometimes important direct benefits; patients may gain access to new methods of therapy not in general use. If there has been no previous available therapy for a given disease, or if therapy has been ineffective, the potential benefit is clear. As an example, studies of new forms of treatment for cancer usually follow so-called protocols; these are carefully defined guidelines that govern the use of new forms of therapy and provide as much information as possible about the risks and benefits of the new drug. Without the new therapy, the patient might well die. Patients terminally ill with advanced heart disease were given an opportunity for a heart transplant when it was still an experimental procedure and not available to them except as research subjects. A similar opportunity, heart-lung transplant, is now being offered to patients with pulmonary hypertension.

Often the potential benefits do not accrue to the individual patient. Patients participating in a study may be serving as the controls—either they are not treated with the proposed intervention or they may be given a placebo. Patients are sometimes asked to take drugs not in order to treat their disease but to study the way the drug is handled by the body. No benefits to the patient are apparent and, if the patient has an adverse reaction to the drug, he is harmed.

We have said that existing safeguards for human subjects are often insufficient, but can we do better? Suppose, for example, that each experimental human subject had access to an ombudsdoctor. Such an arrangement would increase the likelihood that consent would be fully informed, that the patient understood the known risks and benefits and was carefully instructed to detect early adverse effects, and, in general, to safeguard his own best interests. The ombudsdoctor could be selected for his expertise in the area under study, but he would have no interest in the outcome of the study beyond the best interests of the patient.

Balancing the Objectives

It is true that to impose additional requirements for the safeguarding of patients would make the performance of research more difficult. The risk of adding yet another barrier to the performance of clinical investigation is that the rate and amount of research would be reduced. The benefit would be in increased safety for the patient.

We have repeatedly indicated that many of the limitations inherent in medicine are related to deficiencies in the accumulation of patient data. We have maintained that iatroepidemics could largely be prevented by appropriate clinical trials; that the hazards of surveying normal populations could be decreased by performing more clinical trials; and that the uncertain basis of much of current medical practice could be made more secure by appropriate clinical trials. How would this be practical if, at the same time, clinical trials were made more difficult by restrictions designed to increase patient safety?

The conflict between individual patient safety and the requirements of medical progress is a singularly modern development of a more general and ancient puzzle: How to reconcile the welfare of the individual with the needs of the group or, in classic terms, the rights of the individual versus the needs of society. No entirely satisfactory resolution for this universal dilemma has yet been found. It is not surprising that we lack an easy answer to this special case. Given sufficient attention and support, the seemingly opposite goals of more patient safety and a wider use of clinical trials could probably be reconciled. The absolute minimum requirement for continued medical progress is that patients continue to volunteer as participants in clinical studies. It seems reasonable to hope that more informed participation by patients in experimental studies might accelerate, rather than inhibit, the accumulation of worthwhile data.

There are some things you, as a patient, should do. It is imperative that you know as much as possible about your personal role in a research project before agreeing to participate. Read the consent forms carefully; question anything that is not clear to you; and ask for any additional information you feel you need. If possible, ask the advice of your own personal physician, or consult an ombudsdoctor, should one be available to you. If you need more time to collect information about the study, ask for it. Don't hesitate or be too shy to ask the important questions: What are the benefits for me? What are the risks for me? Why are these studies important for other people? How significant are the goals of the study?

Evoke the Golden Rule. Ask the doctor soliciting your participation if he himself would participate in the study under similar circumstances. If you are acting for a member of your family, ask if the doctor would permit members of his own family to participate. Physicians are honorable people and both of you will benefit by this dialogue. If a picture of the study develops that is more disturbing than you anticipated, don't be ashamed to pull out. If you are too ill to make judgments for yourself, have someone in the family assist you.

If you can find it in yourself to do so, try to keep an open mind about participating in studies that may not be of direct benefit to you. To contribute to the progress of medicine and to the welfare of others can be satisfying, but it is *your* decision to make.

14

Peddling the Pedestal

As medical care is increasingly converted into a business, or industry, its practitioners pursue the goal common to all business—profit making. Some individual doctors or groups of doctors operate largely as entrepreneurs and many hospitals operate as money-making ventures. Like all successful entrepreneurs, doctors and hospitals devise ingenious schemes for increasing revenue.

The Doctor as Entrepreneur

Let us look at some examples. One Southern California city has attracted a distinct oversupply of pediatricians. Increasingly, children are admitted to hospitals under the care of two doctors, rather than the customary single pediatrician. The first, the referring pediatrician, is usually a general pediatrician; the second is a specialist in the major area of disease for which the patient is admitted. This dual sponsorship allows both doctors to bill for their services on a daily basis without technically engaging in feesplitting. The specialist is thus not limited to a consultant's fees. Recently, this practice has been extended; three rather than two doctors share the patient and collect three separate fees.

Competition for share of the market has made for jurisdictional disputes between groups of doctors competing for control of a given area of medical testing or care. One current brawl involves government reimbursement for laboratory testing under Medicare. The American College of Pathologists (ACP), which represents clinical pathologists who traditionally run laboratories in hospitals, sued the federal government. The basis of the suit was as follows: Pathologists have customarily collected two separate fees from the federal government for Medicare patients—one, from funds paid to the hospital, as salary for the running of the laboratory; and one as direct payment for "professional services to individual patients." The federal government sought to restrict payment to the sum paid the hospital, and in truth, clinical pathologists provide little or no direct patient services.

The pathologists admitted in court that most clinical pathology procedures "do not require in-person involvement at the time the test is run." But they insisted that the pathologist does play two roles. First, the pathologist must "see that the technical procedures are run with sufficient detail and quality." Second, the pathologist must "be in a position to answer questions put by the general physician who has general care of the patient." They claim that everything that occurs in a clinical laboratory is part of the practice of medicine. Most of this rationalization is hogwash. The clinical pathologist is double-dipping. Only in his direct activities as a pathologist does he provide a needed patient service.

The view point of the pathologists is strongly opposed by a group representing laboratory technicians, who "seek to develop and preserve an environment in which all who offer their services in the clinical laboratory marketplace can do so fully and in competition with others who purport to offer the same services." This is clearly a battle for control of the marketplace and for money. In the opinion of the technicians, pathologists are trying to maintain a closed shop. They are correct.

Competition for patients has intensified among doctors as a result of three factors: *(a)* There are too many doctors, and the disparity between supply and demand is increasing. Doctors are professionally maldistributed; many specialties in medicine are heavily overstaffed—general surgery is one example. *(b)* Doctors are geographically maldistributed. Large cities attract more doctors than small communities. As a result, the competition is fiercer in larger cities, although as the absolute number of doctors grows, even small towns and rural areas tend to have more doctors than are needed. *(c)* As the number of available patients per doctor becomes smaller, the temptation to do more to each patient grows out of economic pressures, even in the absence of other pressures.

Radiologists vie with cardiologists to determine who will perform coronary arteriograms (x-rays of the coronary arteries). Radiologists and neurosurgeons vie to see who will perform CAT scans of the brain. Pathologists and lung specialists vie for the fees collected from the measure of blood gases. Anesthesiologists vie with pulmonary doctors for control of intensive care units. Each contending group claims special expertise in the area contested. Each group pushes its claim on the basis of concern for patient care. Although the question of money is not raised, the conclusion is inescapable—whoever wins the argument pockets the money.

Marketing Strategies

Like any organization with a product to sell, medicine must attract the customer. At a recent meeting of the American Medical Association, a discussion of marketing techniques revealed that doctors are making increased numbers of house calls. This is an instructive example. The increase is apparently not a response to a perceived need to improve patient care; it is a response to increased competition for patients.

During the past 20 years, the unwillingness of doctors to make house calls has evoked strong public criticism. The medical establishment rejected much of the criticism as undeserved, arguing that a doctor can do little at a patient's home, that to care for extremely ill patients at a hospital rather than at home is in the patient's best interests. Now, the AMA reports that, apparently as a result of economic pressures, more doctors are willing to make house calls. If their major concern is the welfare of the patient, they might be expected, rather than limiting the discussion of house calls to their effectiveness as a marketing device, to consider such questions as: What illnesses could best be handled at home? What equipment should be carried on house calls? How long should the doctor attempt to treat the patient before referring the patient to a hospital? For acute and critically ill patients, the use of paramedical personnel specially trained in providing care under field conditions might help more patients than would a major return to house calls by doctors.

A recent example of aggressive marketing is reported in the medical literature. (This episode is so incredible that you might want to read the details yourself.) A letter addressed to the editor, *New England Journal of Medicine* (1983, vol. 309, p. 1194.) by D. Webb reports that a patient came to a clinic carrying with him the results of a test, a carotid artery ultrasound examination. This is a noninvasive test that uses sound energy to determine the patency of the arteries supplying the brain. The test showed that "the right carotid artery was narrowed by 50–70 percent." The patient was worried about his disease and came to the clinic. As the patient had no symptoms suggesting that his carotid arteries were abnormal, the clinic doctor asked why the test was performed.

The explanation was that several self-styled doctors had brought portable equipment to his apartment building to solicit requests for the test. The patient had insurance and thought he might as well have the test performed. The bill was $800, to be paid in part by Medicare and in part by private insurance. He was not given a one-year free subscription to a magazine of his choice as a bonus. Of course, the clinic doctor may have been the victim of a "joke." Or perhaps the purvey-ors of the test were confidence men posing as doctors, rather than vice versa.

If you have any question about the extent to which medicine has converted to a business, look at the section labeled "Physi-cians" in the yellow pages of your telephone directory. One medical group invites you to fly to Southern California for a hair transplant, a face-lift, or the cosmetic surgery of your choice—and promises to refund your round-trip air fare. A medical center offers an array of treatment, from biofeedback to hypnosis, for an even greater array of complaints—from headaches to sexual and mental problems. If you prefer a more traditional approach, you are invited to drop in at any of several no-appointment-necessary clinics and medical offices; your Visa, MasterCard, or personal check will be happily ac-cepted.

The Hospital as a Business

Hospitals are even more aggressively involved in business practices than are individual doctors. A hospital director notes that there is a lag in admissions to the hospital on Fridays; patients preparing for surgery on Mondays are admitted on Saturday or Sunday. In order to fill the empty beds on Friday, a lottery is organized. Patients are encouraged to enter on Friday by the possibility of winning two free tickets to Hawaii.

Proprietary hospitals—hospitals either privately owned or belonging to a corporation and whose acknowledged objec-tive is to make money—are flourishing economically. In gen-eral, proprietary hospitals make more money than nonpro-prietary hospitals. One explanation for this difference is that proprietary hospitals are better run: Centralized purchasing, modern business practices, and efficient use of hospital staff generate more profit. But a careful study failed to confirm this theory. Rather, it appeared that the proprietary hospitals had rediscovered Sutton's Law. Willie Sutton was a famous bank robber. When asked why he robbed banks, he replied in amazement, "That's where the money is." Proprietary hospitals make more money because they charge higher prices than nonproprietary hospitals for the same service.

A certain hospital charges $137.00 for a panel of chemical tests; most of these are not essential for the overwhelming number of patients, but they are routinely performed. The total cost to the hospital of running the tests is $3.50. A commercial laboratory charges $5.00 for the same panel and makes a substantial profit. The patients are overpaying for a service of dubious value. The cost of a bottle of salt solution in this hospital is a bargain. The hospital charges only $47.00 for administering a bottle of salt, the actual cost of which is $6.00.

The same hospital increases prices by approximately 20 percent one year. This increase is not proportionate to the rate of inflation or determined by other obvious economic factors. The hospital is attempting to raise large amounts of money for its own building program, and the patients are involuntarily contributing to it.

This hospital takes its marketing seriously. The administration organizes a planning session for the heads of hospital departments (physicians and non-physicians). An outside financial expert begins by indicating that questions concerning the maintenance of high standards of patient care will be considered out of order. In his view (he is not a doctor and can barely distinguish a patient from a dollar bill), the law of the marketplace takes care of the problem of quality of patient care: If you don't offer quality care, you will lose your customers.

Many American hospitals still operate as so-called nonprofit organizations. To do so provides major tax and other financial benefits, as well as permitting the hospital to solicit contributions from the public. The economic benefits accrue to the hospital administration, some doctors on the staff, and the sponsoring institution, rather than to stockholders—as they do in a proprietary hospital. Little trickles down to the public. The drive for profits is as strong in the not-for-profit hospital as it is in the proprietary hospital. This has adverse effects on patient care, because it encourages practices based on profitability rather than on direct concern for patient welfare.

As the amount of money to be made in medicine has increased, health care has attracted "carpetbaggers" who bring the laws of the marketplace to the hospital in a naked form. Not all medical administrators are carpetbaggers, but their number is growing. One such, while addressing a distinguished group of medical school doctors, informed them, "You better get out and take their patients away." "Their" referred to the private doctors in the same community. No salesman in a used car lot could have been more explicit. The "town versus gown" battle for business between medical school doctors and private doctors is being waged in many communities.

The Impact of Business Practices on the Doctor's Image

How have patients responded to the growing trend to convert medicine into a commercial enterprise or a trade? There has been surprisingly little erosion of the public image of the doctor as an unselfish humanitarian who seeks to help mankind. This image is in part sustained by the many doctors who continue to practice in a largely altruistic way. Some of the continued support derives from the general view of our society that there is nothing wrong with making as much money as possible. Some stems from unawareness of the magnitude of economic abuses found in medicine. And some undoubtedly stems from cultural lag—most patients simply do not recognize that economic motives may influence clinical management.

Entrepreneurial approaches increase potential risks to patients in a number of ways. Excess testing is promoted to increase revenue. You have already learned about the hazards of excess testing. The performance of invasive procedures is encouraged because these bring in even more revenue: A gastroenterologist can charge perhaps $50.00 for a routine office visit lasting one hour; but if he uses a tube to visualize part of the gut (endoscopy), he is paid several hundred dollars for perhaps a 20-minute procedure. A routine examination of the chest does not produce much revenue, but if the patient is bronchoscoped—a tube is inserted in the airways to visualize the inside of the bronchial tube—the payment is many times greater. As a result, bronchoscopy is performed in many more patients than is warranted.

Surgical procedures have built-in economic incentives, and it is probable that these prompt some unnecessary surgery. Economic rewards unquestionably account for some of the enthusiasm for periodic checkups, multiphasic screening, and extensive testing of normal subjects.

Most of this drive for increased revenue acts at an unconscious level. The doctor usually does not deliberately set out to make more money by performing extra or unnecessary remunerative studies. But there is no doubt that extra or unnecessary studies are ordered, especially in hospitalized patients. Doctors who use the hospital facilities more aggressively make more money for the hospital. They are implicitly encouraged to make extensive use of the various services offered by the hospital.

One might expect the exalted image of doctors to suffer a sharp decline unless they change their economic practices. It seems ironic that medicine, usually quite defensive when criticized, largely ignores the criticism provoked by its entrepreneurial behavior. Apparently unwilling to donate its pedestal without compensation, medicine may actually be peddling it, unknowingly, for money.

The Effort to Contain Costs

In recent years, strong pressure to contain the cost of health care has come from groups outside of medicine—from the federal, state, and local government, consumer groups, insurance carriers, and experts who specialize in medical economics. A number of proposals for reducing the costs are already in the process of implementation, among them a plan for so-called "hospital caps." A hospital is paid a fixed fee per patient per day by external providers; this covers all costs, including room and board, laboratory tests, x-rays, all procedures, and doctors' fees. The hospital then allocates the money to its various internal cost centers.

What will be the impact of this on patient care? Reducing payments for tests will undoubtedly cut down the amount of testing. Not only will unnecessary studies be reduced in number, but necessary ones may be reduced as well. The risk is that in selecting the studies to be performed doctors will be influenced by cost; the cheapest studies may be done rather than those that might be best for the patient. Who will have authority to decide on the distribution of available money? Almost certainly, individuals quite removed from direct patient care and, for the most part, not doctors. Of course, hospital caps do not have to work this way, but unless the plans are specifically structured to protect patient care they almost certainly will.

Another proposal establishes preferred provider organizations (PPOs). Insurers pay medical costs only to those selected health care providers that deliver health care at relatively low costs. Medical care is not homogeneously excellent; the cheapest provider is not necessarily the most competent provider, and the quality of patient care may suffer.

The impact of basic changes in economic practices on the quality of medical care remains to be seen. A decrease in medical costs will not automatically insure the best possible medical care. Protecting the quality of care should be a prime consideration in any planning. This consideration has been largely overlooked.

Several things seem obvious. One is that the poor and disadvantaged will bear the brunt of any deterioration in the quality of health care. Another is that the savings will be less substantial than predicted, because they will be swallowed up in the administrative costs of enforcing new systems. Still another is that no one, including the planners, can predict the impact of these changes on the quality of health care. This should be of concern to you.

As an individual patient, what might you do to minimize any detrimental effects of economic factors on your health care? Avoid doctors unless you are truly ill and avoid hospitalization unless necessary—suggestions that have already been made in other contexts. Do not flinch from the explicit recognition that medicine is increasingly practiced as a business. If medicine is a business, you are a customer and you have the right to question and negotiate charges—with doctors, hospitals, insurance companies, and other third parties. But remember that you are more than a consumer; you are also a patient. Ideally you are entitled to the best care at a fair price.

Finally, you should remember that present plans for changing the economic basis of medicine do not contain specific provisions for ensuring an adequate quality of care. You may want—to the extent that your circumstances permit—to use your influence to help correct this critical oversight. Local committees can influence the way hospitals are run. City, state, and federal legislation can affect hospital practices. Congressmen and senators should be made aware of the needs and wishes of their constituents regarding health care. These matters are your legitimate concerns as a citizen.

15

The Patient's Rights
and Responsibilities

Your rights as a patient are inseparable from your responsibilities as a patient. You have the right and the responsibility to

- Be specifically informed about the important details of your care.
- Make an informed choice from among the alternatives available to you.
- Actively participate in your management.

Patients and doctors still question whether the patient should exercise these rights. The answer is an unequivocal *yes*.

As the cost of medical care has risen, the patient's rights as a consumer are increasingly recognized and the need to keep patients from wasting their money is stressed. I am more concerned with keeping patients from wasting their lives. In this chapter I have therefore tried to give you some explicit direction for exercising the rights and responsibilities that will help you and your doctor to fulfill his job description: *To optimize your chances for a happy and productive life.*

You may appreciate the advantages of greater patient involvement in clinical management, but at the same time you may have reservations about your ability to contribute in a way that improves the outcome of your care. You may feel that you don't know enough. True, you cannot write a prescription, but you can become an informed patient by gathering information about your disease from all the sources available to you, including your doctor.

You may fear that the doctor will resent your intrusion. Indeed he may. If he cannot accept your partnership, it may be necessary for you to find a doctor who will. You may be unwilling to take responsibility for altering his decision and thus affecting the outcome. No decision, yours or his, is infallible, and it is your life.

A Good Example to Follow

A recent encounter I had with a husband and wife in a hospital reaffirmed my belief that the patient and the patient's closest family can and should take responsibility.

A 44-year-old woman, mother of three, was dying of heart failure caused by primary pulmonary hypertension (high blood pressure of the blood vessels of the lung). As her condition became more desperate, the proposals for managing her disease became more frantic.

Her doctors suggested that she undergo an open-lung biopsy, because it might reveal the cause of the pulmonary hypertension. Her husband, a clear-thinking and far-sighted person, questioned her doctors: What was the probability that the results of the lung biopsy would help his wife? The doctors equivocated but ultimately gave an honest and accurate answer. There was essentially no chance that the lung biopsy would lead to effective treatment. How much pain and suffering might his wife endure as a result of the surgery? Again, he received an honest answer. Some additional pain and suffering were inevitable. And was there a risk that his wife might die as a result of the surgery? To be sure, there was a risk of death. Patients with his wife's illness not uncommonly die even from mild forms of stress, let alone surgery on the lung.

Having obtained the answers to his questions, the husband refused to allow a lung biopsy. The wife agreed. This episode is remarkable in several respects. One is the perceptiveness of the husband. He is not a physician, but he was able to analyze his wife's problems precisely and accurately. In fact, he intuitively performed a superb risk-benefit analysis and concluded that the proposed biopsy was essentially all risk and no benefit. He was willing to accept responsibility for a decision that went contrary to the advice of the doctors. Not many lay people would be willing to act in this way.

How can we explain the position of the doctors? It is not that they were badly trained or anxious to operate at the expense of the patient's welfare. On the contrary, they were highly motivated, good humans. But they were frustrated at their inability to influence the course of the wife's illness favorably. They watched her dying day by day and wanted to do something, however ill conceived.

Most situations are not this clear-cut, but this husband's behavior is a good model for you to follow. Can you imagine yourself as a mother telling your pediatrician how to care for your child? You may not easily see yourself in this role, but your minimum responsibility is to be fully informed about what is being planned and to exercise your best judgment as to whether it is appropriate.

Some Explicit Questions to Ask

How can you meet your responsibilities as a patient or as a close relative of a patient?

- Remember that your doctor is not your adversary and don't let your relationship develop into an adversarial encounter. Ideally, you are partners in an enterprise that has larger implications for you than for him.
- Remember that your doctor is not a god and relate to him as a fellow human.

You have both the right and the responsibility to ask the doctor a series of questions:

- Why are you doing this test (or tests)?
- What are the risks?
- What are the benefits?

· What is the rationale for the treatment you propose?
· What are the risks of the treatment?
· What are the benefits of the treatment?
· What will you do if the treatment does not work?

When tests are planned, you might request answers to these seven questions:

· Is the test technically satisfactory? [Many are not, but are nevertheless performed.]
· How safe is the test?
· What is the sensitivity of the test? Most simply, what is the percentage of false negatives? [See glossary.]
· What is the specificity of the test? Most simply, what is the percentage of false positives? [See glossary.]
· How accurate is the test? [The true negatives plus the true positives divided by the total number of tests.]
· What is the general patient effectiveness of the test? [What does the medical literature have to say about the effectiveness of this test in promoting better decisions in patients who have your problem?]
· What is the specific patient effectiveness for you? [How does the doctor expect to use the information in managing your illness?]

Putting these questions to your doctor will usually not only prove useful to you in making an informed decision; it will help *the doctor* in planning and carrying out your care.

Finally, you have the right to reject those portions of the doctor's plan that do not seem to you to be in your best interests.

Doctors differ widely in training, experience, skills, and character—and in their capacity for compassion. All doctors are not created equal; they are not equally well trained nor do they practice equally well. Patients should recognize this fact and attempt to obtain the best possible care.

If you decide that an advanced or unusual form of management is necessary, you will want to select the doctor and institution most experienced in that modality. Remember that the period immediately following the introduction of a new modality is associated with the highest morbidity and mortality. Eventually, we hope, not every medical institution will try to offer every procedure; only designated centers will provide specialized procedures. Until that day arrives, try to avoid places and doctors who are still in their learning phase.

Sometimes the "best" is dictated by circumstance. For example: Only two or three medical centers perform heart-lung transplantation; a limited number offer certain kinds of cancer therapy; and only a few provide some specific types of radiologic treatment.

Apply the Golden Rule: Ask your doctor where he would go or whom he would consult were he in your situation. Don't be satisfied by partial or evasive answers.

Try to select a doctor who is willing and able to enter into the kind of relationship you want—a doctor who can be sensitive to your wishes and needs, with whom communication will be a dialogue rather than a monologue, and who will have as his explicit goal the best possible solution of your medical problem.

The Role of the Ombudsdoctor

Now, of course, there are many situations in which your lack of medical expertise will make you feel appropriately insecure about interpreting the doctor's answers, let alone deciding what to do about them. For those times, you might well adopt a measure I have proposed in several different contexts in this book, and that is to use an intermediary as your representative and advocate—an ombudsdoctor.

The function of the ombudsdoctor would be to advise you and to represent you in health care encounters so that you can make the most rational and informed choices possible. As your advisor, he should have no ego investment in your decision and no economic stake in the planning of your medical care. He should be a doctor who has kept up with modern medicine so that he can explain the full range of options available to you. He should also have broad contacts in the medical community so that he can help you find the best doctors available to treat your particular illness and the best places that offer the necessary treatment.

The ombudsdoctor should be a physician willing to devote the time and attention your specific problems demand. He should know enough about the various branches of medicine to guide you through encounters with specialists. Ideally, the ombudsdoctor should know enough about your family and circumstances to enable him to understand you and your needs.

Finally, the ombudsdoctor should act as a translator of words and ideas for you. Too often the doctor who is treating you is not an adequate source of information. This may sometimes be a result of an unwillingness or inability to communicate, but beyond those possibilities there are at least two specific barriers to communication between doctor and patient. One is that doctors speak a separate language, "Doctorspeak." Like "Newspeak," the language described by George Orwell, Doctorspeak is more apt to obscure than to illuminate meaning. Doctors' jargon is not usually understandable to patients. For example, a disease whose cause is not known is referred to as "idiopathic." It sounds very learned, but it merely means "the cause is not known."

Here is an example of Doctorspeak offered by a fellow physician. A patient complains of pain in the back of the neck. After the patient is examined, he is informed that he is suffering from cervical spondylosis. Translated into English, this means that there is something wrong with the spine in the patient's neck—hardly a major addition to what the patient already knew, but it sounds impressive.

Other barriers to the patient's understanding exist: The concepts, ideas, and specialized information that constitute the doctor's knowledge about given areas of medicine may be difficult for the patient to assimilate. The ombudsdoctor could assume responsibility both for translating from Doctorspeak and for summarizing the information the patient needs in order to make informed choices.

The choices that patients must make can be unbelievably complex. In Chapter 6, I described a new drug, cyclosporin-A, as particularly effective in preventing rejection of new organs in human transplantation. The drug, you will remember, has its risks; it can cause lymphoma, cancer of the lymph system. The patient must balance the potential benefit of successful transplantation against the potential risk of cancer. It now appears that the effects of cyclosporin-A can be reversed. After cancer develops, the withdrawal of cyclosporin-A may cause regression (subsidence) of the cancer; it will, of course, also increase the risk of transplant rejection. The patient may now have to repeat a complicated risk-benefit analysis. In such circumstances, the usefulness of an ombudsdoctor is unquestionable.

Several questions arise: Should all doctors be ombudsdoctors? The answer is no; this is not practical. Doesn't the description of the ombudsdoctor fit the typical family doctor? The answer is perhaps, but that was a long time ago and under other circumstances. The kindly family doctor belonged to a time when medical care was much simpler; much less could be done to and for patients; and the choice of available treatments and procedures was much narrower. If he attempted to function in the old way today, the general practitioner would not be able to do what is now required of him—to keep up with a very complex and rapidly developing discipline.

Is this proposal contrived and unnecessary? No. It is not reasonable to expect doctors who are highly skilled technically and highly specialized—and such doctors are essential to the medical care system—to make your overall interests as a distinct and individual patient their leading priority. Nor can the busy general practitioner or family doctor usually qualify for the role. Much or most of medical care is delivered by teams of doctors. In a highly developed, complex medical system, this is inevitable. What these teams often lack is someone to represent the patient. The ombudsdoctor would do that.

You may think that the characteristics of an ombudsdoctor as outlined above are simply those you expect to find in your doctor. If so, you have a set of criteria to use in selecting *"your* doctor."* You may say that what has been described is no more than what your doctor already does. If you have such a doctor, then you are very fortunate; you already have your ombudsdoctor.

How Patients Increase Their Risks

There are some things that even an ombudsdoctor cannot do for you unless you exercise both your rights and your responsibilities. I have repeatedly emphasized the risks inherent in the medical system because most patients are unaware of them. My analysis would be incomplete if I failed to point out those risks that patients create for themselves.

If the partnership with your doctor is to work, you must cooperate with him. Doctors complain, with some justice, that patient compliance with instructions is often poor; sometimes, admittedly, the instructions may be unclear, but noncompliance is most frequent when the medicine or other treatment has unpleasant side effects.

Patients are often overly impressed by aggressiveness; they judge the doctor's competence by the intensity or amount of testing he pursues: A high degree of intensity and a huge number of tests are equated with medical excellence. If the testing makes use of impressive gadgetry—complex electronics, computer control, or radioactivity—the patient is inclined to believe that the best of modern medicine is being practiced and that doctors who do not offer these refinements should be shunned.

Many doctors assert that they are forced to overtest and overtreat as a defense against accusations of malpractice. The number of malpractice suits has increased in recent years and the price of malpractice insurance has skyrocketed. As a result, doctors claim, they are now required to practice "defensive medicine." Defensive medicine seems to mean that the doctor performs every test that can conceivably be justified in the context of the patient's problem. A hospital administrator has estimated that one-third of medical costs stem from attempts to forestall malpractice suits. Although the figure seems grossly exaggerated, it points to an important reality.

Of course, many malpractice suits are valid, the doctor having been, in fact, negligent. However, in our system of law, anyone can sue anybody at any time and frequently does. This lends itself to abuse; plaintiffs—and the lawyers who represent them—can expect large settlements when they win. Perhaps a system of arbitration, rather than litigation, for settling claims would be more equitable. But, in any case, the specter of a malpractice suit affects the practice of doctors who might otherwise avoid unnecessary testing in the management of patients.

A Definition of Malpractice

To understand malpractice, you must know what a doctor does *not* have to do to meet standards of legally acceptable medicine.

A doctor is not required to achieve a successful outcome in individual patients. Such a guarantee would be impossible to fulfill. Whatever the skills and experience of the doctor, many illnesses simply cannot be brought to a successful outcome (see Chapter 4). In fact, the doctor expects to be paid (and has a legal right to be paid) whether he has treated you successfully or not.

Doctors do not have to restrict treatment to measures that have been adequately tested. They are permitted to introduce new practices in medicine without adequate trials of the risks and benefits. They are permitted to try completely untested methods of practice, especially when the circumstances of the patient's illness seem to warrant the trial.

Society grants the doctor privileges denied other professions. The doctor is not restricted to those areas of medicine in which he has been specifically trained. Theoretically, a psychiatrist could practice cardiac surgery. Doctors and medical students are permitted to use patients for whom they are caring as appropriate objects of study.

A doctor does not have to be correct to be innocent of malpractice. The required standard is that his medical practices conform to the minimal levels of care as practiced in the community. This interesting principle implies that it is acceptable for a doctor to be wrong as long as all other doctors in the community are wrong in the same circumstance. Doctors participating in iatroepidemics (the subject of Chapter 8) are presumably protected because, at the time, most doctors were equally guilty of the errors that caused the epidemic. Collective malpractice in medicine is usually not considered to be malpractice at all.

Media Medicine

Too often, patients allow "media medicine" to shape their ideas and expectations of medical care. A great volume of health-related information flows through the media. The average magazine reader and television viewer in the United States can easily be convinced that he or she is fully informed about the latest developments in almost every disease that might eventually afflict him, his family, or friends.

Fortified by "facts" gleaned from the media, the patient may be inspired to unrealistic expectations. If the reality falls short of his expectations, he may demand more aggressive treatment. To satisfy the patient, the doctor may be forced to overtest and overtreat, thereby creating additional risks for the patient. If he judges it best not to meet the patient's demand, the patient may shop around for another doctor who will overtest and overtreat him.

When illness strikes, an informal network of relatives, friends, and acquaintances will often form for the purpose of volunteering and exchanging medical information—often information gleaned from magazine and newspaper stories, TV programs, perhaps even novels and soap operas. Each new development that surfaces anywhere is detected by this well-meaning network and relayed to the patient. Family and friends barrage the patient with articles, clippings, and phone calls; they urge a change of doctors, a change of treatment, a visit to one medical center or another. These interventions almost never help.

The public has a right to information on medical progress and change, and for this they must turn to both the medical establishment and the media. Doctors should cooperate to keep the public well informed, and the media has a legitimate right and even responsibility to provide information that it considers helpful or newsworthy. But it can be taken as a general principle that media information cannot be more valid than that provided by medical art and science at the time. If, as you have learned, even the medical literature leaves much to be desired in terms of authenticity, certainly nonmedical sources cannot provide more valid—and often provide less valid—information. When the media trumpets a new discovery, beware.

This is not to say that media medicine cannot be valuable. For example, a national television program presents a report on research on paraplegics. The use of computerized, regulated, electrical stimulation of muscles to enable patients whose legs have been paralyzed by spinal cord injuries to walk is being tested. The program is skillfully done. The doctor in charge of the research is reserved and modest in his claims.

The patients are enthusiastic and well informed about the research studies. The viewer is left with admiration for the indomitable spirit of these gravely handicapped people.

The media in this instance have provided a real service. The research is being done at a small, relatively unknown medical school. Research on paraplegics is not one of the glamor fields in medical research; many doctors, paraplegic patients, and their families may not be aware of the new possibilities displayed on the program. At the very least, the program provides them with some realistic hopes for the future.

This standard of excellence is not always achieved. Doctors sometimes release material that lends itself to sensational and inaccurate interpretation by the media. They may be prompted by ego, by a desire for personal or professional advancement, and, occasionally, by a hope of improving their chances for research support.

Acquired immune deficiency syndrome (AIDS) is very much in the news. A relatively new disease in its presently observed form, it is usually found in homosexuals but also in some Haitians, and in some patients receiving transfusions or blood products. AIDS has received wide public attention because it is associated with a high death rate (perhaps 50 to 70 percent of those affected) and because it is of grave concern to an important minority—the homosexual population.

AIDS kills patients by reducing their immunity to a wide range of infections; it is also associated with an unusual form of cancer, Kaposi's sarcoma, which, it is speculated, could be caused by decreased resistance to cancer. The possibility of contracting AIDS raises deep fears in almost everyone and, understandably, even deeper fears in homosexuals.

The cause of AIDS is unknown (there are claims that it is caused by a virus), and no known therapy has been found to be effective for the primary disorder. One *theory* is that it is caused by an abnormality of T-lymphocyte cell function. T-lymphocytes are a cell type important in the defense mechanisms of the body against various infections and other disturbances. An investigator makes the national newspapers and television by announcing a breakthrough in AIDS. The breakthrough consists of a new test for T-lymphocyte function that *perhaps* could help in the diagnosis. Even if it were verified as a diagnostic tool, there is no way in which the test can be applied to the treatment of AIDS. To describe this development as a breakthrough is a gross exaggeration. (Undoubtedly, many claims for breakthroughs in AIDS will continue to be reported.)

In this instance, the media have accurately reported the claims of the investigator; it is the investigator who has extravagantly overemphasized the importance of the finding even as a diagnostic tool, let alone as a breakthrough. This kind of act may unintentionally mislead large numbers of people.

Not infrequently, however, the media contribute to the inaccuracy of medical reporting. It is the reporter's job to enhance the newsworthiness of any material; he will often press the interviewee to commit himself further than he had intended —to make a greater claim for a putative discovery than should be made. After persistent questioning, the interviewee may finally capitulate and exaggerate the importance of his findings.

Certain buzz words seem to stimulate the media to an excess of enthusiasm. Anything to do with cancer or heart disease gets a high priority. The media have announced any number of breakthroughs in these two diseases over the past 20 years; most have come to nothing. Smoking and nutrition are favorite topics. A charismatic doctor will receive more extensive media coverage than a sober, everyday doctor. Unfortunately, there is little relation between the media appeal of a doctor and the accuracy of his information.

The media can hardly be expected to evaluate critically the content of medical material. Suppose the media critically evaluated political, economic, social, or cultural information; they could shake the very fiber of American life. My aim is not to criticize the media. The point I want to stress is rather that those who accept media information uncritically are putting themselves at risk.

The public is not sufficiently aware of how superficial and premature much of the medical "news" is—and how often it is unverified. There is an interesting misconception that a conspiracy exists within the medical establishment to prevent major advances in medical science from being used in medical practice. That such an impression should arise is understandable, but it is unwarranted. There are not many secrets in medicine or medical science; it is unlikely that important new breakthroughs will escape the attention of most doctors. Actually, the reverse is true. Thanks to a highly effective but uncritical system of medical communication, useless and harmful "advances" are sometimes adopted. If effective approaches in medicine are sometimes not readily adopted, do not take it as evidence of a conspiracy or of an inadequate system of communication. The fault lies rather in the limitations of the medical care system.

A Realistic View of Doctors

Two accurate statements that doctors could make—and with great frequency—are "I don't know" and "I was wrong." But one doctor seldom makes these statements to another and almost never to a patient. Obviously, doctors feel that such statements would undermine their authority with patients. It is the rare patient who can accept either of these statements without becoming unraveled emotionally or setting out on a frantic search for a doctor who will be more (even if inappropriately) confident that he is invariably right. Every doctor is frequently uncertain and frequently wrong. As a patient, you must accept this as a reality and not use it as a basis for judging your doctor.

If you have taken this book seriously, you will view your relationship with your doctor as a partnership in which you are the informed patient, he the trained professional. Your acceptance of him as a partner implies a measure of trust. If you want to know more, ask him. If you disagree with him, tell him. Any doctor worth his fee welcomes an informed patient.

Back to Basics

In the first chapter I set forth the rationale for this book in the form of three assertions:

1. There are serious flaws in the basic processes by which diagnostic and therapeutic measures are introduced and used in medicine.

   The bulk of the book has been devoted to an analysis of the medical system that gives rise to these flaws, to evidence of their existence, and, to their effects.

2. Many of the flaws in the basic processes by which diagnostic and therapeutic practices are introduced and used in medicine can be corrected.

   In pointing to the flaws in the medical system I have throughout the book made recommendations for change. These are summarized and expanded in an appendix following this chapter.

3. Potential or actual patients can reduce the risks and increase the benefits of their medical care if they are familiar with the flaws in medicine.

   My purpose in writing this book has been to alert you to the risks and benefits of medical diagnosis and therapy. In this chapter I have made explicit recommendations for increasing the benefits and protecting yourself from the risks. Do you as a patient or potential patient have a stake in these proposals? Indeed you do. These are matters of life and death.

Epilogue

I have throughout this book emphasized, as I promised I would in the first chapter, the risks of medical care. As the book neared completion, I participated in the care of a patient. I want to tell you her story as a way of reminding you of the benefits of our medical system.

This 85-year-old woman suffered a rupture of an abdominal aneurysm, which is a swelling of the main artery in the body, the result of weakness in the aortic wall. Despite her age, she wanted reparative surgery. She was competent to make such a decision—it was *hers* to make—and her daughter supported her choice. As she was being brought to the operating room, the aorta gave way completely and most of her blood gushed through a hole in the aorta into her peritoneal cavity. Her blood pressure dropped to zero and her heart stopped.

Her doctors restarted her heart and gave her transfusions of 16 pints of blood. They replaced the diseased part of her aorta with a plastic graft. The next morning, she was a reacting, thinking human being. Her life had been saved almost miraculously, although temporarily.

The story does not have a happy ending. After an initial period of improvement, the burden of her 85 years and the trauma of the overwhelming hemorrhage, the cardiac arrest, and the surgery took their toll. Her kidneys, lungs, and heart failed. This multi-organ failure depressed the function of her brain and she lapsed into an irreversible coma.

As it became obvious that her condition was hopeless, her daughter and the doctors conferred. They decided that the major goal of her management should be to shield the patient from additional trauma and suffering and that they would therefore provide only minimal life support. When she was removed from a ventilator her breathing stopped and within minutes she was dead.

This patient's care was exemplary. Even the process of her dying was well managed. Our medical system, although imperfect, is capable of extraordinary achievements. More important, the system is capable of being changed for the better. That is the single most hopeful fact.

Appendix: Recommendations for Changing the Medical System

This is a book for patients, not for doctors. The changes recommended can be effected only with the support of the medical system itself, but an informed patient is an asset to that system. As a patient you influence your doctor by your attitude, by your expectations, and by the degree to which you take responsibility for your own treatment. The greater the interest on the part of patients, the more aware the medical system will become of the need to correct its flaws.

Reform the Training of Medical Students

Unless far-reaching changes are made in the training of medical students, the next generation of doctors will repeat the errors of previous generations.

Medical training should lead to the conviction that the primary goal for every doctor is to achieve an improved outcome for patients; that diagnosis, medical education, and scientific investigation are secondary to the well-being of the individual patient.

A substantial part of the medical curriculum should be devoted to an in-depth analysis of the limitations of medicine and the limitations of doctors. The tentative nature of much of medical knowledge should be explicitly emphasized, and medical students must be taught to evaluate the medical literature critically. The application of risk-benefit analysis to every aspect of patient care should be a major component of medical training.

A frank recognition of the deficiencies in medical knowledge would create that atmosphere of humility essential to every doctor's realistic self-appraisal. It would also serve to weaken the hierarchical structure that is now the rule in medicine and make for a greater closeness among all the members of the medical care team—doctors, nurses, paramedics—and for their greater efficiency as a team.

To fulfill these urgent needs, medical students must be taught

- How to arrive at a balanced evaluation of new technologies and information if they are to avoid glaring errors implicit in the too rapid introduction of untried approaches.
- To be alert to the causes of iatrogenic episodes and iatroepidemics. Measures designed to minimize these dangers to patient welfare should be explored.
- To avoid dogma by recognizing that much of medical knowledge is not fixed but constantly changing, and that they have the right and the responsibility to change patient management once it has been established that the old approaches are useless or harmful.
- A critical but respectful approach to basic medical science. They should be thoroughly grounded in the application of basic science to medical care and understand that the models used by basic science are often not relevant to patient care.
- Above all, how to listen to patients and to respect both their wishes and their opinions.
- Not to usurp those decisions that belong to the patient, foremost among them being decisions that determine the lifestyle of the patient and the intensity of treatment.

To reduce the surplus of physicians, which leads to added risks for patients, the number of students admitted to medical schools should be decreased.

Expand Clinical Trials

A properly conducted clinical trial is the most reliable method for determining the risks and benefits of a procedure or treatment. Among the measures that would make possible the expansion of these trials to the degree required for adequate protection of patients are these:

- A substantial share of the necessary financial support should be provided by the federal government as an investment in the health of its citizens.
- A center for stimulating and organizing clinical trials could be established under the umbrella of the National Institutes of Health.
- The majority of these trials should be conducted at medical schools because *(a)* much of the required expertise is available at these institutions, *(b)* participation would provide excellent training for medical students, and *(c)* it would enable medical schools to get out of the health care "business" by providing an alternate source of funds for the school. One of the most corrupting influences on young doctors is the commercialization of the medical school—its use of marketing methods and advertising and its economic competition with the private sector of medicine. (Private donors should withhold support from medical schools that sacrifice academic goals for economic advantage.)
- Some clinical trials should be conducted in community hospitals because the patient population and the nature of the care provided at these hospitals are more representative of the community. The outcome of such trials would therefore be more directly applicable to the general community.
- International sponsorship of clinical trials would produce benefits greater than those that can be achieved by any single country.

Perform Only Specifically Relevant Diagnostic Procedures

In place of its present shotgun approach to diagnosis—the performance of numerous studies, many of which are irrelevant to the specific medical problems of the patient—medicine should adopt a much more selective and specific approach. Many of the studies routinely performed on patients do not contribute to their well-being and may harm them.

Set More Rigorous Criteria for the Screening of Normal Subjects

No major screening effort should be introduced until its efficacy, sensitivity, specificity, and accuracy have been determined by a clinical trial. In particular, such trials should be designed to disclose the likelihood of false-positive findings and the fate of false-positive patients, as well as the long-term hazards to all subjects screened.

Voluntary health organizations should take the leadership in sponsoring these careful preliminary trials. The public should be alerted when organizations sponsor mass screening not based on acceptable clinical trials.

Assure Adequate Support for Basic Medical Science

Basic medical research, an inefficient and frustrating but compelling human activity, is the only mechanism that can prevent medicine from remaining frozen in its present unsatisfactory state. Adequate financial support and resources must be allotted for basic medical research by government, industry, foundations, and the general public.

Reduce the Number of Doctors and Hospitals

There is an oversupply of doctors in the United States. As a result, patients are overdoctored; this is bad for patients.

Society must pay for this overdoctoring; this is bad for society. Doctors are thrust into sharp competition with each other; this is bad for doctors, and bad for patients, whose best interests may be sacrificed for the economic survival of the doctors.

The same considerations apply to hospitals. There are too many hospital beds and patients are overhospitalized. This is bad for patients, for society, and for hospitals, which must compete with each other for business.

Change the Attitude of Medicine Toward Its Errors and Its Critics

The opportunity to acknowledge medical errors, to learn from them, and to correct them requires a less defensive and more open attitude within medicine than currently exists. This kind of honest exchange can flourish only in an atmosphere that encourages constructive criticism and the open acknowledgement of systematic errors by their originators. Above all, it requires a system that insures a rapid decay of harmful practices.

The Feasibility of These Suggestions

Are these proposals practical? Economically, yes. Ten percent of the funds now expended each year on unnecessary or harmful medical care would be more than enough to support these suggestions.

Are these proposals politically, socially, and scientifically feasible? Probably, if there were general public agreement that the measures proposed are necessary.

Glossary

accuracy The number of accurate results divided by the total number of tests performed.

acquired immune deficiency syndrome (AIDS) A disease usually found in homosexuals, and also in some Haitians and patients receiving blood products, in which a number of normal defense mechanisms against infections and cancer are depressed.

acute A disease manifestation that develops quickly; as contrasted with *chronic*.

adenine arabinoside (ara-A) A drug used to treat herpes encephalitis.

adrenalectomy Surgical removal of the adrenal glands. A discredited form of treatment for high blood pressure.

adult respiratory distress syndrome (ARDS) A form of lung failure caused by acute injury to the lung.

Alzheimer's disease A leading cause of sequential loss of memory, confusion, and dementia primarily found in the aged.

amebiasis An infection caused by amebae, which may involve the liver.

amphotericin B A drug used to treat various fungal infections.

angiogram An x-ray showing the vascular system after the injection of radiopaque material.

ankylosing spondylitis A form of arthritis in which the joints in the vertebral column become immobile.

anorexia Loss of appetite.

antacids Drugs used to neutralize acid in the stomach.

antibiotics   Drugs derived from fungi and bacteria and used in the treatment of infections.

anticoagulants   Drugs that prevent blood clotting.

aorta   The main artery, arising from the left ventricle of the heart, from which the arteries supplying blood to most tissues of the body arise.

aortogram   An angiogram of the aorta.

artificial lung   An experimental apparatus that supplies oxygen to and removes carbon dioxide from patients with abnormal lung function.

asbestosis   A group of diseases caused by exposure to asbestos.

asthma   A group of diseases in which the bronchial tubes become intermittently narrowed. Its leading cause is frequently an allergic reaction.

atropine   A drug used for various purposes such as treatment of hyperactivity of the GI tract and rapid heartbeat.

barium enema   The instillation of barium into the colon followed by x-rays for the purpose of detecting abnormalities in that organ.

basic research   Research that concerns itself with the mechanisms of various biological processes.

Behçet's syndrome   Characterized by ulcerations in the mouth and genitals and abnormalities of the eye and other organs.

biguanidines   A group of drugs, formerly administered for the treatment of diabetes, that produced severe complications in some patients.

biologic variation   The tendency of individual subjects to react differently to the same alteration. For example, the same dose of a drug administered to two closely matched subjects may result in different responses.

biopsy   Removal of tissue from a living body in an attempt to establish a diagnosis.

blood types Immunologic groups that characterize the red blood cells of various individuals.

bone marrow The pulpy substance in bone that is the site of manufacture of many blood cells.

bradytachyarrhythmias Heart rates that are too slow (bradycardia), too fast (tachycardia), or irregular (arrhythmia).

brain death Permanent cessation of brain function.

brain stem death Permanent cessation of function of the lower part of the brain, which controls such activities as breathing and heart action.

bronchitis Infection or inflammation of the bronchial tubes.

bronchoscopy The insertion of an instrument into the airways for direct visualization of the inside of the bronchial tubes and sometimes for obtaining a biopsy of these structures. Almost certainly vastly overdone from the viewpoint of patients.

buddy system The practice of one doctor's referring his patients to another doctor because the second doctor is his friend.

cancer A group of diseases in which cells undergo unregulated growth and potential invasion of other tissues.

cancerguiltia Feelings of guilt when one, or member of one's family, develops cancer. These feelings are never objectively warranted.

cancerphobia Excessive fear of cancer.

carbon monoxide A poisonous gas that can cause disability or death if inhaled at a suitably high concentration.

carcinoma in situ (CIS) Localized cancer cells that do not invade other tissues for long periods of time. There is some reason to believe that these localized cells may occasionally disappear spontaneously.

cardiac arrest Stoppage of the heart.

cardiac catheterization Insertion of a hollow tube into the various chambers of the heart for the purpose of measuring pressure, amounts of oxygen and carbon dioxide, and the volume of blood being expelled.

cardiac output   The volume of blood expelled by the heart each minute.

cardiac pulmonary edema   Excessive fluid in the lung caused by heart disease.

cardiogenic shock   Decrease in blood pressure and cardiac output caused by direct injury to the heart muscle.

cardiopulmonary resuscitation (CPR)   Restoration of ventilation and cardiac pumping by external maneuvers in the event of cardiac arrest or cessation of breathing.

cardiovascular failure   Failure of the heart or vascular system to function normally.

carotid artery   The principal artery on each side of the neck, which carries blood to the brain.

carotid artery ultrasound examination   A test for determining whether the inside of the carotid artery is normal.

carpetbagger (medical)   A person who is not an integral part of the health care system who invades it primarily for the purpose of making money.

catheter   A hollow tube that is positioned in various organs either for the removal of fluids or for the performance of various measurements.

cervical spondylosis   Any abnormality of the part of the backbone that is in the neck.

cervical stenosis   A narrowing of the cervix of the uterus (the entrance). One of the complications of conization.

chemotherapy   The use of various drugs in the treatment of cancer.

chloramphenicol   An antibiotic drug used for the treatment of various infections.

chronic   Present for a long time; as contrasted with *acute.*

class 3 Pap smear   An abnormal Pap smear that is not frankly malignant and is consistent with dysplasia.

claudication   Limping or pain resulting from a decrease in the blood flow to the legs.

clinical management   The sum total of diagnostic and therapeutic efforts that a doctor undertakes on the patient's behalf.

clinical research   Direct studies of disease processes, usually in patients.

clinical trial   A study of the efficacy of a given form of diagnosis or treatment that can be used to estimate the risks and benefits of a procedure or treatment. Interestingly enough, despite its central importance in medicine, the term is not listed in medical dictionaries.

coccidioidomycosis   A fungal infection particularly common in the southwestern United States.

colonoscopy   Insertion of an optical system into the colon for the purpose of inspecting the inside and also for obtaining a biopsy of suspicious areas.

colposcopy   The insertion of an optical system for the visualization and biopsy of the cervix.

compliance   The patient's obedience to the doctor's orders. Note the use of the term "orders" to indicate the doctor's advice or instructions. In other contexts orders are issued by a superior to a subordinate.

Computer Axial Tomography (CAT scan)   A powerful diagnostic approach that views various organs in the body by a complex x-ray system.

congenital   A disease with which one is born. The disease is usually, but not always, inherited.

congenital hypothyroidism   Lack of adequate amounts of thyroid hormone; a condition present at birth.

conization   Removal of a cone-shaped part of the cervix or uterus for the purpose of biopsy or treatment.

consensus panel   A panel of experts who issue a report in a given area after achieving a consensus decision.

consent form   A form given to a patient for his signature to record the agreement of the patient to participate in a given study or treatment. These forms are often so complex that even physicians and attorneys have difficulty interpreting them.

control group   A group that is either not given a form of treatment or diagnosis or is treated with a placebo in a study of a test or a form of treatment.

coronary artery disease   Disease of the arteries supplying the heart, usually caused by narrowing of these blood vessels.

coronary bypass surgery   Surgery that bypasses narrowed portions of the coronary arteries in an attempt to normalize blood flow to the heart.

coronary care unit (CCU)   A separate unit in the hospital in which patients who have had heart attacks, or are suspected of having had heart attacks, receive care.

Creutzfeldt-Jakob disease   A brain disease found in middle-aged and older adults, resulting in abnormalities of behavior, emotional responses, memory, reasoning, and vision and by peculiar jerking movements of the muscles. The disease progresses with great rapidity, so that deterioration may be seen from day to day. Said to be invariably fatal.

critical care medicine   A branch of medicine that deals with critically ill patients.

curettage   The scraping of tissue from a cavity, such as that of the uterus.

cyanosis   A bluish discoloration of the skin and mucous membranes caused by various abnormal states.

cyclosporin-A   A drug used to inhibit the rejection of transplanted organs by the body.

cytomegalic virus infection   A virus infection that may produce no symptoms or may produce pneumonia or other abnormalities.

defensive medicine   Medicine practiced to decrease the possibility of malpractice suits.

dementia   Physical deterioration of the brain.

detail man   An agent of a pharmaceutical house who visits doctors in hospitals to dispense drugs and sometimes advice.

diagnostic efficiency The number of accurate diagnoses made by a given test, divided by the total number of tests performed.

diagnostic nihilism The belief that diagnostic tests should not be performed. A term that may be used to characterize individuals who insist that the risk-benefit ratio of a test should be established before it is widely employed.

diethylstilbestrol (DES) A synthetic female sex hormone used as an estrogen replacement and formerly misused in an attempt to prevent miscarriages.

Doctorspeak The jargon that doctors use in communicating with each other and often with patients.

double-dipping Accepting two payments for one piece of work.

dysplasia Alteration in size, shape, and organization of adult cells; commonly found in cells from the cervix and believed by some to be a precancerous stage.

edema Excess fluid in the tissues.

elective surgery Surgery that is not immediately lifesaving or that can be performed at the discretion of the surgeon or patient.

electrocardiogram The record produced by the electrical activity of the heart.

embolism The blocking of a blood vessel by a clot or foreign material brought to the blood vessel by the circulation.

emergency surgery Surgery required quickly, often for lifesaving purposes.

encephalitis, herpes Inflammation of the brain caused by the herpes virus.

encephalitis, viral Inflammation of the brain caused by a virus.

endoscopy A test in which the inside of an organ is visualized through an appropriate optical system.

false negative A result that indicates that a patient does not have a given disease or abnormality, which, in fact, he does have.

false positive A finding that indicates that a patient has a given disease or abnormality, which, in fact, he does not have.

femoral vein ligation Tying off the major veins of the leg in an attempt to keep clots from reaching the blood vessels of the lung.

fiberoptic tube An optical system used in various forms of endoscopy.

fibrocystic disease Numerous cysts found in the breasts of women. Previously regarded as a precursor of cancer, it now appears that, for most women, this is not true.

fluoroscopy Visual observation of the inner structures of the body by means of x-ray shadows projected on a fluorescent screen.

galactosemia An inherited deficiency of an enzyme leading to mental retardation, cataracts, and abnormal liver and kidney function.

gastrojejunostomy Surgical connection of the stomach to a part of the small intestine.

geriatrics A branch of medicine dealing with the aged.

glaucoma A group of eye diseases characterized by an increase in eyeball pressure.

glue ear A childhood disease in which a thick fluid collects behind the eardrum. Evidence exists that there is a high incidence of false positives leading to a large number of unnecessary operations.

God Only Knows (GOK) A common outcome of extensive diagnostic workups that lead to no specific diagnosis. The diagnosis may then be said to be, "God only knows."

heart-lung transplantation Removal of the heart and lungs from a brain-dead donor and transplantation into a recipient with terminal lung or lung blood vessel disease.

hemorrhoidectomy Surgical removal of hemorrhoids (piles).

heparin A drug used to prevent clotting.

hepatitis, infectious Inflammatory disease of the liver often caused by virus infection.

hexachlorophene An antibacterial agent used by medical personnel to wash their hands. Absorption of the agent through the skin of premature infants can result in brain damage.

history The initial part of the medical workup, in which the patient describes symptoms, past medical history, and other matters relevant to his illness.

hospital caps Setting a ceiling on the amount of money paid to a hospital per patient per day.

human experimentation committee A local group set up to review proposed experiments on humans for the purpose of protecting the experimental subjects.

hydatoxic lualba A mythical worm that was described as the cause of pre-eclampsia-eclampsia but turned out to be talc from the powder in surgical gloves.

hypertension An increase in blood pressure.

hypothyroidism Diseases associated with deficiencies of thyroid hormone.

hysterectomy Removal of the uterus.

iatroepidemic A plague caused by doctors. An iatro-epidemic consists of a systematic error incorporated into medical practice that results in harm to or death of large numbers of patients.

iatrogenic episodes Accidents that occur to patients during management as the result of individual mishaps. These episodes are not the result of systematic errors and are random in occurrence.

idiopathic Cause unknown.

idiopathic thrombocytopenia purpura (ITP) A rare condition of unknown cause in which the blood platelets (see *platelets*) are deficient in number, resulting in hemorrhages at various sites in the body.

ileal bypass A surgical procedure in which the last part of the small intestine is bypassed to help obese people lose weight.

immune process   The process involved in the resistance of the body to infection.

immunosuppressive   Descriptive of drugs that suppress immunity. Useful in treating various immune diseases and also in preventing rejection of transplanted organs.

in-between surgery   Surgery the necessity of which is not clear-cut; the decision whether to operate or not is difficult for surgeon and patient.

infiltration   Penetration of a tissue by other cells, fluid, or aberrant tissue *(infiltrates)*. Used to describe an appearance on a chest x-ray of abnormal shadows that are not regular in outline.

informed consent   A process by which a patient, having been made as fully aware as possible of the risks and benefits of a given management proposal, agrees to that management. This ideal is seldom attained for a variety of reasons —including the possibility that the doctor himself may not have an accurate idea of the risks versus the benefits.

informed refusal   A process in which the patient, having been fully apprised of the risks and benefits of a given management proposal, decides that he does not want the proposal implemented.

intensive care unit (ICU)   A separate unit in the hospital set aside for the treatment of the critically ill.

intensivists   Specialists in intensive care medicine.

invasive   Descriptive of a procedure in which the body is physically invaded.

invasive carcinoma of the cervix (ICC)   Cancer of the cervix that has spread from its original site and has invaded adjacent tissues.

investigator   The person responsible for initiating a medical experiment.

irreversible   A state of damage so severe that the process cannot be reversed. This does not mean that death of a given organ has occurred. For example, irreversible brain injury means that the brain is beyond recovery from a given injury.

Kaposi's sarcoma A malignancy of the skin consisting of multiple soft bluish tumors. May develop as one of the manifestations of AIDS.

kidney dialysis A form of treatment for kidney failure in which toxic substances are removed from the blood.

lactic acidosis A form of increased acidity of the blood in which lactic acid, a byproduct of normal body metabolism, accumulates.

laetrile A compound containing cyanide said to have anticancer properties, although evidence indicates that this is not true.

leukemia A blood disease in which the white blood cells are abnormal in number and kind.

lithium A chemical element that is highly effective in the treatment of some patients with manic-depressive psychosis.

liver coma Failure of the liver, causing depression of the brain.

lumpectomy Surgical removal of a small cancer of the breast. A form of surgical operation that is an alternative to simple mastectomy or radical mastectomy.

lung scans Tests widely used in attempts to diagnose pulmonary embolism.

lymphoma A cancer arising in the lymph tissue.

malpractice Legally, a failure to meet the standards of treatment or care in a given community. In some states, the standards of care are variable, depending on the training of the doctor whose conduct is being questioned.

mammary artery ligation An operation previously employed for patients with coronary artery heart disease, which proved to be of no value.

manic-depressive psychosis A psychiatric disorder in which periods of excitement alternate with periods of depression. Its exact cause is not known, but there is growing evidence that it is related to a chemical disorder of the brain and may respond to treatment with lithium.

mastectomy   Surgical removal of the breast. May involve removal of the breast (simple mastectomy) or removal of the breast and much of the surrounding tissue (radical mastectomy).

medical system   The sum total of medical knowledge and medical practice generally accepted at any given time.

meningitis   Infection or inflammation of the meninges, the membranes covering the brain and spinal cord.

metastasis   The spreading of disease from one part of the body to another. Usually refers to cancer, but infections may also spread.

metastasizing clone   Single cells in a cancer, which carry the cancer to distant tissues and give rise to metastasis.

metastatic cancer   Cancer that has spread beyond its original site, usually to another tissue or organ.

minor operation   An operation done on someone else.

monitoring   Measuring bodily functions over a significant period of time.

morbidity   The sick rate. When pertaining to diagnosis or treatment, it refers to the number of complications, divided by the number of patients tested or treated.

mortality   The death rate. When referring to a test or treatment, mortality is the number of people who die as a result of the test or treatment, divided by the number who are tested or treated.

muscular dystrophy   A congenital disorder of the skeletal muscles associated with weakness and inadequate muscle function.

myelogenous   Relating to white blood cells.

myocarditis   An inflammatory disease of the heart muscle (myocardium).

myoclonus   Peculiar involuntary muscle contractions seen in a variety of neurologic diseases such as Creutzfeldt-Jakob disease.

necessary surgery The risk-benefit analysis indicates that the operation is likely to increase the happiness or productivity of the patient.

neonatal Newborn; usually up to one month of age.

no code A patient in whom cardiopulmonary resuscitation will not be attempted, even in the case of cardiac arrest or cessation of breathing.

nodule A small bump. For example, a roundish spot on a chest x-ray.

nonsystematic errors Accidental, nonrandom errors inadvertently made in patient care.

nuclear medicine That field of medicine which uses radioisotopes for the diagnosis and treatment of certain diseases.

oat cell cancer A form of cancer of the lung in which metastasis occurs very early.

ombudsdoctor A doctor who serves as the advocate and representative of the patient in medical encounters.

open-lung biopsy A biopsy of the lung obtained through the chest wall.

optical system A tube for insertion in some part of the body and a series of lenses and lights.

Papanicolaou (Pap) smear A smear obtained from the cervix, which is then examined microscopically to determine if cancer cells are present.

paramedics Nonphysicians and nonnurses who provide medical care.

paraplegic Paralyzed in the lower limbs, usually including the sphincters that control the bladder and rectum.

parotid glands A pair of glands located in front of and below the ear that secrete salivary fluid.

pearls Medical opinions, frequently not based on acceptable evidence but pronounced with great authority. Almost invariably highly regarded by the opinion giver and often accepted as being of great value by the recipient.

peer review Judgment passed by experts in a given field on the validity of medical articles, the merit of grant applications, or the value of various forms of diagnosis and treatment.

peptic ulcer   An ulcer in the stomach or duodenum (first part of the small intestine).

pericarditis   Infection or inflammation of the membranes surrounding the heart (pericardium).

perirenal   Describing tissues that surround the kidney.

phenylketonuria (PKU)   An inherited congenital metabolic abnormality that results in mental retardation, neurologic manifestations, dermatitis, and a mousy odor if not adequately treated with a special diet.

physiological age   A subjective estimate of the patient's functional age as compared to his actual chronological age.

placebo   An inert substance given to a control group during the course of determining the effectiveness of a drug or medical intervention. Ideally, neither the patient nor the physician is aware of which is being used—the actual agent or substitute. Occasionally used by doctors for its psychological effect.

plasma   The liquid part of the blood.

platelet   A formed element of the blood important in the process of blood clotting.

pleura   The membranes covering the lung.

pneumothorax   Air or gas in the pleural space.

polyp   A tumor with a stalk, usually arising inside an organ.

potassium intoxication   Adverse effects resulting from too much potassium in the body, usually revealed by higher than normal levels of potassium in the plasma.

preeclampsia-eclampsia   A group of diseases that affect pregnant women, characterized by high blood pressure, decreases in kidney function, and sometimes coma, convulsions, and death.

preferred provider organization (PPO)   A medical group that agrees to provide medical care at discount rates.

premalignant A condition characterized by precancerous changes in cells or tissues.

primary pulmonary hypertension Increases in blood pressure in the blood vessels of the lung; its cause is not known.

proprietary hospital A hospital overtly operated to make a profit for its owners.

prospective study A study in which the ground rules for gathering and interpreting data are pre-set.

protocols A prearranged set of rules for providing various forms of treatment.

psychosurgery Surgery performed for the putative relief of psychiatric diseases whose causes are believed not to result from anatomical disturbances in the brain. Performed on thousands of patients, it left most of them more disabled after the surgery than before. The tragic consequences are vividly depicted in the book *One Flew Over the Cuckoo's Nest* by Ken Kesey.

puerperal fever Childbed fever, a disease that killed thousands of women, now known to be an infectious disease caused by bacteria and frequently spread from patient to patient by doctors with dirty hands.

pulmonary edema Excess fluid in the tissues of the lung.

pulmonary embolism A solid bit of matter, usually a blood clot, carried in the bloodstream from another site in the body and impacting in the blood vessels of the lung.

pulmonary function testing A collection of tests to assess the function of the lung; vastly overdone, as judged by the actual value to the patient.

radioimmunoassay A form of laboratory test for measuring very small quantites of proteins or similar chemicals in the body fluids and tissues. One of the originators was awarded the Nobel Prize for this test although the original work was rejected for publication by a major scientific journal.

radiopaque material A material that obstructs the passage of x-rays, thus producing white shadows on exposed x-ray film.

red blood cells   Formed elements in the blood containing hemoglobin, a protein that combines with oxygen to ensure an adequate supply of oxygen to the body tissue.

regression   Reversion to a previous state. For example, spontaneous regression of a tumor means that the tumor disappears and the tissue becomes normal.

renal failure   Failure of the kidneys.

reproducibility   Consistency of results.

respiratory failure   Failure of the lungs to pick up enough oxygen and to excrete enough carbon dioxide to maintain normal function of the body.

retrolental fibroplasia   Blindness in newborns, usually caused by exposure to excess amounts of oxygen.

retrospective study   Data collected from records and similar sources, in which the conditions of study are not established prior to the data collection. As a result, many errors of interpretation may occur.

Rh negative   Absence of one blood group Rh factor. May result in incompatibility of blood groups between mother and fetus, leading to destruction of the red blood cells and causing abortion or harm to the fetus. Can be prevented by injecting a protein into the mother.

risk-benefit analysis   An analysis assessing the potential risks versus the potential benefits of a given procedure.

salvageable   A blunt term widely used to describe patients who can be returned to a happy and productive life.

screening   The process of applying a test or tests to a large population in an attempt to pick up disease at an early stage.

senile dementia   Physical deterioration of the mind during old age. The most common cause appears to be Alzheimer's disease.

sensitivity   The number of true negatives divided by the number of false negatives plus the number of false positives.

Shiller test   Painting the cervix with an iodine solution in an attempt to detect areas with cancer. Has been proven to be grossly unreliable, but is still used by some doctors.

sigmoidoscopy The insertion of an optical system for visualizing the rectum and a portion of the colon.

sleep apnea A group of disorders in which the patient has prolonged periods of cessation of breathing while asleep.

specificity The number of true positives divided by the number of false positives plus the number of false negatives.

spondylosis Any abnormality of the backbone.

status thymaticus A mythical childhood disease; doctors treated infants with x-rays to prevent it, thereby causing a high incidence of cancer of the thyroid in the treated children.

stool guaiac examination A test for blood in the stool.

superficial femoral vein ligation A worthless operation for preventing pulmonary emboli that was widely performed.

Sutton's Law Willie Sutton was a famous bank robber; when asked why he robbed banks, he replied with what has become a classic rejoinder: "That's where the money is." Sutton's Law is widely practiced by many hospitals and doctors.

Swan-Ganz catheter A tube "floated" into the blood vessels of the lung and used for making various measurements. Despite its widespread use, it is useful on only a small number of patients and can harm patients.

sympathectomy Surgical removal of part of the sympathetic nervous system. Formerly used to treat hypertension but now abandoned.

syndrome A group of symptoms or signs which, occurring together, produce a recognizable pattern.

systematic Having a regular and decipherable pattern.

thalidomide A drug taken by pregnant women that produced abnormalities in limbs of the children. It is now said to be of value in the treatment of Behçet's syndrome.

therapeutic efficiency The value of a test in improving the therapy of patients.

therapeutic nihilism The failure to use any therapy in disease. A term that is used to characterize individuals who insist on high standards of validation before a given form of treatment is widely used.

thrombolytic therapy   The use of drugs to dissolve blood clots.

thromboneurosis   Excessive and unwarranted fear that one is suffering from blood clots.

T-lymphocytes   A cell type in the body important in defense mechanisms against various infections and other disturbances.

tomato effect   Discarding a valuable form of treatment because of an inadequate trial. Derived from the shunning of tomatoes as a food in the eighteenth century in North America because tomatoes were thought to be poisonous.

tonometry   Measurement of the pressure within the eye.

transplantation   The process of implanting a donor organ in the body of a recipient.

transplant rejection   Rejection of a transplanted organ by the body of the recipient.

ultrasound   A test in which sound waves are used to outline various body structures.

unnecessary surgery   Surgery that does not optimize the possibility of a happy and productive life.

ventilator   Mechanical apparatus that breathes for the patient.

ventricular premature beats   Extra beats that originate from heart muscle of the ventricles. Occasionally these may be the precursor to a life-threatening disturbance of the rhythm of the heart. Often these beats are harmless.

vital signs   Temperature, pulse rate, blood pressure, and rate of breathing. These are frequently measured in hospitalized patients.

white blood cells   Formed elements in the blood important in body defense mechanisms.

workup   The taking of a history, performance of a physical examination and tests to establish a diagnosis and/or treatment for a patient.

Index

About the Author

Eugene D. Robin, professor of medicine and physiology at Stanford University Medical School since 1970, has distinguished himself as physician, basic scientist, and teacher. Educated at the University of Chicago and George Washington University, where he earned his M.D., Dr. Robin held faculty posts at the Harvard Medical School and the University of Pittsburgh Medical School before coming to Stanford. He has been visiting professor at numerous medical schools in the United States and abroad—among them Harvard, Yale, Johns Hopkins, the University of Pennsylvania, the University of Chicago, and Edinburgh University. Honorary lectureships have taken him in recent years to Ireland, France, England, Scotland, Germany, the Philippines, and Hong Kong.

At Stanford, Dr. Robin teaches medical students, interns, residents, and postgraduate physicians and is actively engaged in the care of patients in both general internal medicine and pulmonary medicine. His scientific research currently centers on molecular genetics; his contributions to research on clinical medicine, marine biology, and cell physiology are recorded in over 200 papers published in scientific and medical journals. As scientist and teacher, Dr. Robin has trained over one hundred young physicians and scientists for careers in academic medicine and science.

A former president of the American Thoracic Society, Dr. Robin has been chairman of the Pulmonary Advisory Committee of the National Heart and Lung Institute and is presently consultant to the National Institutes of Health and to the Veterans Administration. He has also served as consultant to the governments of France and Ireland on scientific matters and on problems in the organization of science, specifically on the relation of basic science to clinical science. In the course of his teaching and his travels, Dr. Robin has tested the ideas in *Medical Care Can Be Dangerous to Your Health* in seminars and in lectures to over 100 audiences of doctors in the United States and abroad.

Dr. Robin's pursuits range into territory not usually visited by physicians. Since 1978, he has taught in Stanford's Freshman-Sophomore Seminar Program; the first three years his subject was Russian literature. In 1980 a lecture tour of Ireland sparked an interest in Irish problems and history, which became the subject for his seminars in 1981, 1982, and 1983.